D1574477

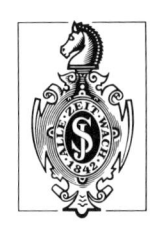

H.-G. Knoch W. Klug

Stimulation of Fracture Healing with Ultrasound

Translated by Terry C. Telger

With 48 Illustrations

Springer-Verlag
Berlin Heidelberg New York
London Paris Tokyo
Hong Kong Barcelona
Budapest

Prof. Dr. Dr. HANS-GEORG KNOCH
Doz. Dr. sc. med. WINFRIED KLUG
Zentrale Hochschulpoliklinik
Medizinische Akademie
„Carl-Gustav-Carus"
Fetscherstraße 74
O-8019 Dresden, FRG

Translator:
TERRY C. TELGER
6112 Waco Way,
Fort Worth,
TX 76133, USA

Translated from the original German edition
Knochenbruchheilung mit Ultraschall
Springer-Verlag Berlin Heidelberg 1990

ISBN 3-540-53674-4 Springer-Verlag Berlin Heidelberg New York Tokyo
ISBN 0-387-53674-4 Springer-Verlag New York Berlin Heidelberg Tokyo

Library of Congress Cataloging-in-Publication Data. Knoch, Hans-Georg. [Knochen-bruchheilung mit Ultraschall. English] Stimulation of fracture healing with ultrasound / Hans-Georg Knoch, Winfried Klug. p. cm. . Translation of: Knochen-bruchheilung mit Ultraschall. Includes bibliographical references. Includes index.
ISBN 3-540-53674-4 – ISBN 0-387-53674-4 (alk. paper)
1. Fractures – Treatment. 2. Ultrasonic waves – Therapeutic use. 3. Wound healing.
I. Klug, Winfried. II. Title. [DNLM: 1. Fractures – therapy. 2. Ultrasonography.
3. Wound Healing. WE 180 K72k] RD 103.U47K6613 1991 617.1'5 – dc20 DNLM/
DLC

This work is subject to copyright. All rights are reserved, whether the whole or part of the material is concerned, specifically the rights of translation, reprinting, re-use of illustrations, recitation, broadcasting, reproduction on microfilms or in other ways, and storage in data banks. Duplication of this publication or parts thereof is only permitted under the provisions of the German Copyright Law of September 9, 1965, in its current version, and a copyright fee must always be paid. Violations fall under the prosecution act of the German Copyright Law.

© Springer-Verlag Berlin Heidelberg 1991
Printed in Germany

The use of registered names, trademarks, etc. in this publication does not imply, even in the absence of a specific statement, that such names are exempt from the relevant protective laws and regulations and therefore free for general use.

Product liability: The publisher can give no guarantee for information about drug dosage and application thereof contained in this book. In every individual case the respective user must check its accuracy by consulting other pharmaceutical literature.

Typesetting: Konrad Triltsch, Graphischer Betrieb, Würzburg
21/3130-543210 – Printed on acid-free-paper

Preface

Every bone fracture requires a certain period of immobilization, sometimes prolonged, in an individual who may otherwise feel completely well. This accounts for the numerous attempts that have been made to accelerate the process of fracture healing. Having worked on this problem for some 25 years, we have found an effective callus-stimulating factor in the piezoelectric effect of ultrasound. Now, thanks to the far-sightedness of Springer-Verlag, we are able to present this clinical experience, backed by experimental data, in book form. We know from the specialized literature that researchers in other countries lately have begun to report on similar experience with ultrasound. Although we have practiced ultrasound therapy in Europe for many years, the political situation has made it impossible for us to publish on the international level. Springer now redresses that situation by enabling our results to be presented to an international readership.

I express thanks to my colleague Dr. med. W. KLUG for the experimental work, to Mrs. CHR. UHLMANN for typing the manuscript, and above all to the reader at Springer-Verlag, Dr. U. HEILMANN, for contacting me at a time when an insurmountable barrier still divided our land. Her constant willingness to help, her promptness, and her congenial cooperation are most gratefully acknowledged.

H.-G. KNOCH

Contents

1	Introduction	1
2	Methods of Clinical Application	3
2.1	Indications and Contraindications	3
2.2	Technique	4
3	Clinical Results	9
3.1	Radial Fractures	9
3.2	Scaphoid Fractures	13
3.3	Metacarpal Fractures	14
3.4	Phalangeal Fractures	17
3.5	Forearm Fractures	17
3.6	Humeral Fractures	23
3.7	Clavicular Fractures	24
3.8	Malleolar Fractures	25
3.9	Tibial Fractures	25
3.10	Femoral Fractures	29
3.11	Patellar Fractures	30
3.12	Calcaneal Fractures	31
3.13	Metatarsal Fractures	33
4	How did we Come to use Ultrasound?	34
5	What is Ultrasound?	40
5.1	Physical Parameters	40
5.2	Characteristics of Ultrasound Therapy	42
5.3	Types of Ultrasound	42
5.4	Mechanisms of Action	43
5.5	The Piezoelectric Effect in Bone	45
5.6	Ultrasound Conductivity	49
6	Animal Experiments	52
6.1	The Rabbit as an Animal Model	52
6.2	Experimental Method	52
6.3	Statistical Evaluation	53
7	Effect of Ultrasound on Fracture Callus	54
7.1	Radiographic Studies	54
7.2	Strength Tests	56

7.3	Histologic Studies, Scanning Electron Microscopy	59
7.4	Bone Scintigraphy	60
7.5	Angiographic Studies	65
7.6	Biochemical Studies	66
7.7	Total Mineral Analysis	75
7.8	Sequential Polychrome Labeling	77
7.9	Temperature Measurements	79
7.10	Summary of Findings	80

Appendix on Instrumentation 81
    High-Frequency Instruments 81
    Low-Frequency Instruments 86
    Safety Aspects 86

References 89

Subject Index 95

1 Introduction

We may define a traumatic bone fracture as a wound of the osseous tissue. Varying amounts of time are required for a wound to heal – less in soft tissues, more in bone. In the past 100 years a great many attempts have been made to accelerate the process of fracture healing. Unlike the healing of soft-tissue wounds, fracture healing requires the immobilization of entire body parts, prolonged inactivity, and the associated prolonged suspension or restriction of normal work and recreational activities.

As early as 1965, following an exhaustive analysis of previous attempts to expedite fracture healing, we found that the piezoelectric effect of ultrasound in bone tissue exerts a stimulatory effect by its ability to accelerate callus formation. In later years it was discovered that the same effects could be produced with electrical energy. It is important to note, however, that the basic mechanism of piezoelectricity underlies the effects of both modalities. Based on experience to date, we may say that callus formation cannot be induced by pharmacologic, mechanical, hormonal, biological, or alimentary means, but only by physical processes. To substantiate this, it must be shown that the bone tissue that forms during the course of fracture healing is equivalent to healthy bone in every respect – clinically, radiologically, histochemically, histologically, angiographically, and in terms of its mineral composition and metabolism. In addition, the new bone must form at a significantly earlier stage in fracture healing than occurs with conventional fracture treatment. There is clinical experience to substantiate this temporal difference.

Proof of the callus-stimulating piezoelectric effect also must be provided along with evidence that the effect is produced both by ultrasound energy and by electrical energy.

The phasic process of fracture healing is well known and need not be detailed here. Regardless of technical progress in fracture management, every fracture must be reduced and immobilized. Absolute immobilization of the fracture site is of fundamental importance. In terms of physical callus stimulation, it does not matter whether a fracture is treated operatively or conservatively.

What are the properties that characterize normal bone tissue? What is expected from healthy bone as an organ? A fracture destroys the bone tissue in the sense that it destroys its function as an organ. The structure, mineralization, and strength of bone can vary depending on the age and sex of the individual. The essential goal of fracture treatment is to restore the original structure, mineralization, and strength of the fractured bone quickly and effectively. By comparing a healthy bone with a healed fracture, taking into account clinical, radiologic, physical, and biochemical parameters, we can confirm that the fracture has healed uneventfully within a certain period of time, and that the bone again exhibits normal osseous structure and can resume its role as a fully functioning organ. This can be proven only by comparison with control groups. After years of studying the pertinent literature, extensive animal experimentation, and more than 20 years' clinical experience in the stimulation of fracture healing in patients treated operatively as well as conservatively, we are able to advance the following theses:

1. A stimulatory effect with an acceleration of bone healing can at present be achieved only by utilizing the piezoelectric effect in bone. This effect can be produced by both ultrasonic and electrical energy.
2. The treatment of a fracture with ultrasound can shorten the course of healing by 30%–50%.
3. Sudeck's dystrophy does not develop in fractures treated with ultrasound.
4. Postfracture rehabilitation is simplified by the shortened period of immobilization, which permits an earlier return to work.
5. Ultrasound therapy is safe, simple, causes no complications, and can be administered in all settings.

2 Methods of Clinical Application

Based on studies in laboratory animals, the known phases of fracture healing, and the properties of ultrasound energy, we have been able to formulate specific indications, regimens, and techniques for the ultrasound stimulation of fracture healing during the past 20 years. Our clinical experience is based on results in 2500 patients who were treated at three medical institutions under virtually identical conditions.

2.1 Indications and Contraindications

Both acute fractures and delayed unions are amenable to ultrasound therapy. For acute fractures, all the known rules of fracture treatment apply: reduction, immobilization, exercise, and follow-up. In terms of response to ultrasound therapy, it does not matter whether the fracture is treated conservatively or by open reduction and internal fixation. Ultrasound treatments are started between the 7th and 10th days after the injury, following organization of the fracture hematoma.

Under certain conditions almost any fracture can progress to a nonunion, regardless of the mode of treatment. The development of a nonunion is always preceded by the stage of delayed union or, as we call it, "delayed callus formation." We use this term clinically to denote a failure in the timely development of callus tissue, with radiographs showing little or no evidence of callus formation following the usual period of immobilization or internal fixation. Untreated, delayed callus formation inevitably progresses to nonunion and therefore should constitute a warning sign for the physician, compelling him to choose between further immobilization or operative intervention. Ultrasound therapy is particularly useful in cases of this kind, for it can stimulate bridging of the fracture site and promote bony union.

Like any therapeutic modality, the ultrasound treatment of bone has certain contraindications. These include systemic febrile states, nonunions, acute osteomyelitis, and primary and secondary bone malignancies.

To date, ultrasound has not been used in the treatment of cranial fractures, spinal fractures, or pelvic fractures.

We do not feel that ultrasound is contraindicated for fractures of the ribs, sternum, or toes, but we no longer treat these cases ultrasonically because the average course of healing is sufficiently short to cause the patient little inconvenience or discomfort.

2.2 Technique

The intensity of the applied ultrasound is from 0.1 to 1 W/cm^2 and the average duration of a single treatment 5 min, depending on the location of the fracture (see Chap. 3). Acute fractures receive a course of 10–20 treatments, delayed unions more than 20 treatments administered on alternate days. Most acute fractures are treated daily, skipping weekends, although small bones may be insonated on alternate days.

We use either a small ultrasound transducer with a radiating area of 1.4 cm^2 or a large transducer with a radiating area of 6.4 cm^2, depending on the area to be treated and the size of the cast window.

We no longer use purely static insonation, where the applicator is held stationary on the skin. We move the transducer very slowly in a linear (stroking) pattern, a spiral pattern, or very often in a circular or sinusoidal pattern (see Sect. 5.4 for exceptions).

The ultrasound may be applied directly over the fracture site or indirectly over the proximal or distal bone fragment (Figs. 1–3). It also may be applied transarticularly, in which case twice the usual intensity is used. Indirect insonation can also be applied through a prominent part of an internal fixation device, such as the head of a Küntscher nail (Fig. 4). In this case the intensity is reduced by one-third. Distant or indirect insonation is made possible by the excellent acoustic conductivity of bone tissue and internal fixation material (Figs. 5 and 6).

A neutral, liquid oil is used to couple the transducer to the skin. The coupling medium should be warmed slightly before applying. Any break in acoustic contact between the transducer and skin is indicated by an audible and/or visible signal from the ultrasound instrument.

Another way to couple the transducer to the skin is by immersing both the target and the applicator in a water-filled receptacle. This method is suitable for fractures stabilized by rigid internal fixation or immobilized in a waterproof cast. Our favorite type of receptable is a ceramic basin with no metal parts (stopper, etc.). Degassed water is used, and small air bubbles should be wiped from the skin surface. The water should be warmed to body temperature. Also, the treatment basin should be of adequate size. If the basin is too

Fig. 1. Direct insonation (small transducer) of a scaphoid fracture through a windowed cast. Absolute immobilization is not disturbed

Fig. 2. Fracture of the proximal third of the humeral shaft, immobilized in an abduction splint and insonated indirectly (small transducer) through a distal window in the cast

Fig. 3. Distal radial fracture immobilized by a forearm plaster slab and insonated indirectly (large transducer) from a proximal site over the radial head

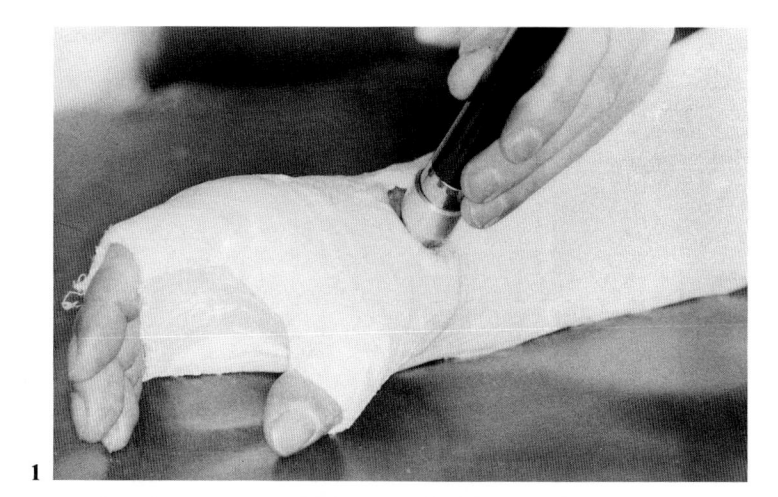

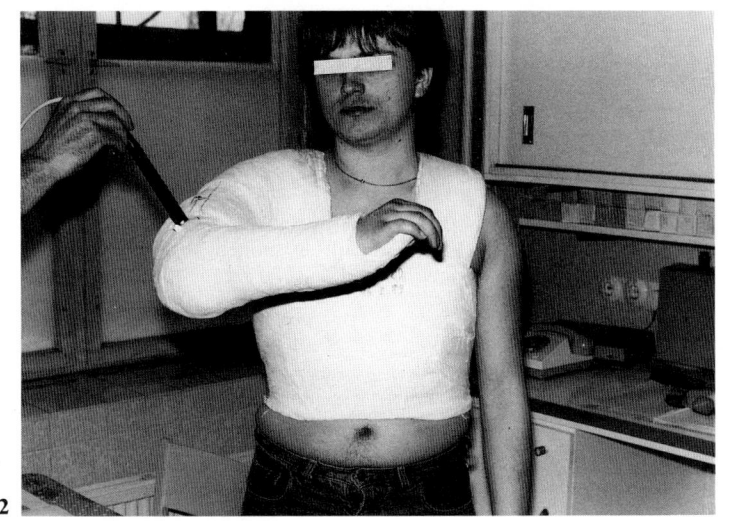

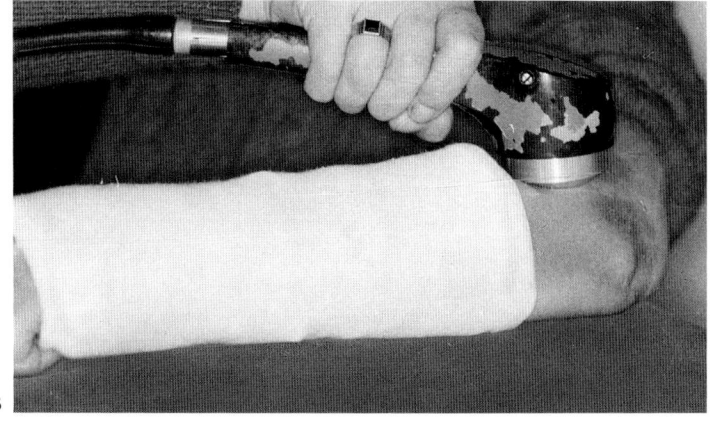

Technique

1

2

3

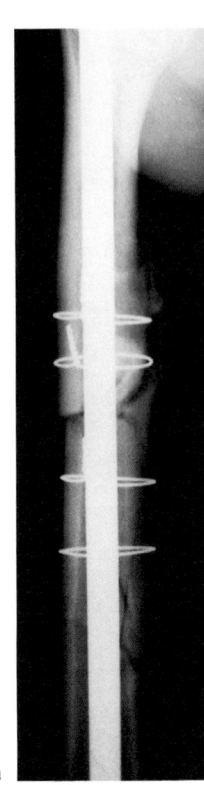

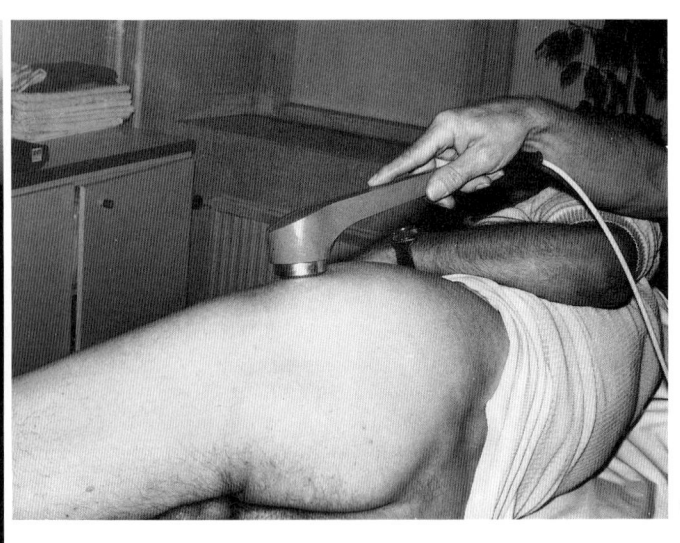

Fig. 4. a Femoral shaft fracture following internal fixation with a Küntscher nail. **b** Indirect insonation over the head of the Küntscher nail and the greater trochanter (large transducer)

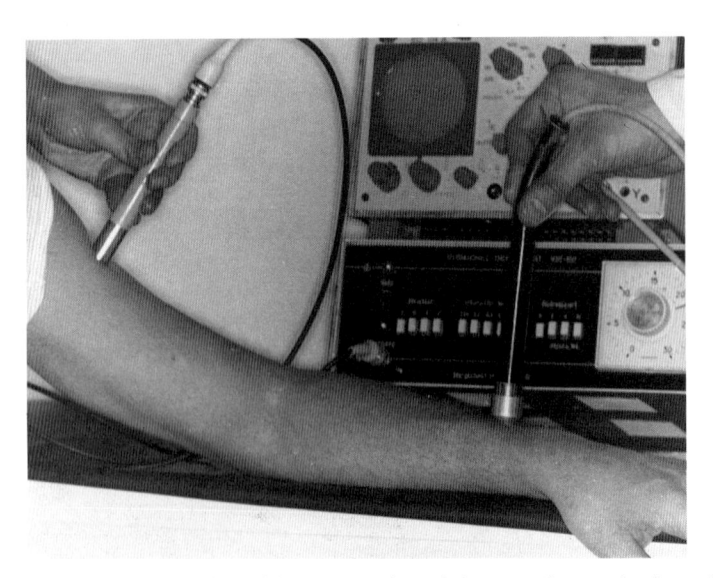

Fig. 5. Demonstration of the propagation of ultrasound waves in tissue. Energy transmitted into the wrist can be detected and measured in the upper arm, and vice-versa

Technique

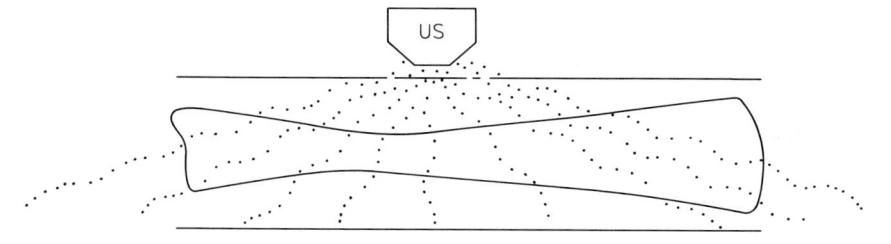

Fig. 6. Schematic diagram of ultrasound propagation in bone tissue

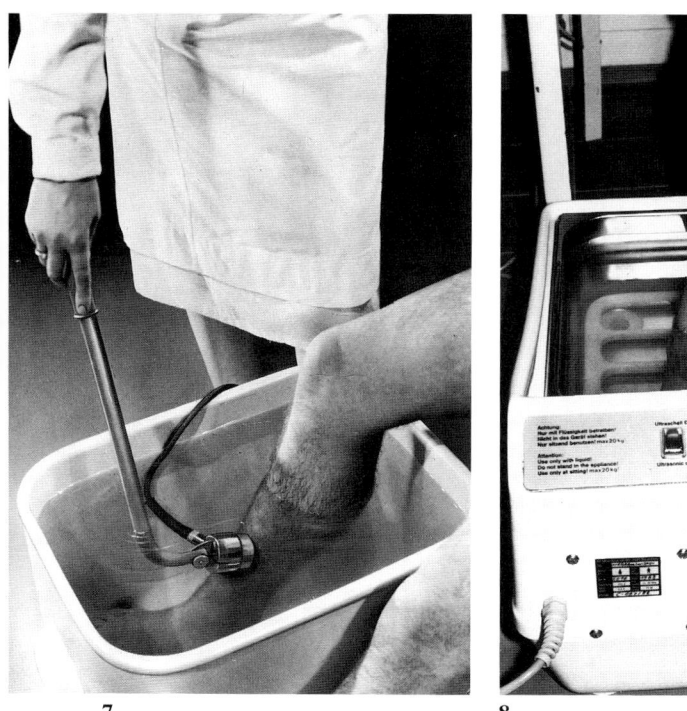

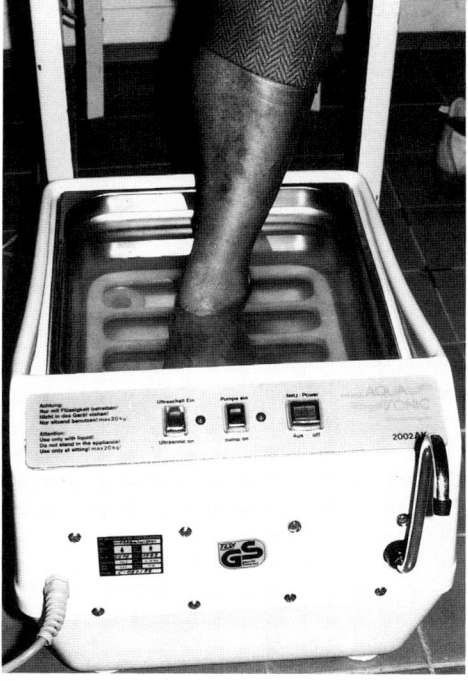

Fig. 7. Tibial fracture stabilized by rigid internal fixation and directly insonated in a water bath

Fig. 8. A metacarpal fracture with soft-tissue ulcerations is treated with low-frequency ultrasound in a water bath (Aqua-Sonic)

small, sound reflected from the walls will produce a nonuniform treatment field due to the mixing of continuous and standing waves. The distance between the transducer and skin should be 1–2 cm; the transducer is moved as described above (Fig. 7).

The same therapeutic effect can be achieved with low-frequency ultrasound (Fig. 8). In this case the transducer is mounted beneath a metal basin into which the affected extremity is immersed. The scheduling and duration of treatment are as previously described. High- and low-frequency ultrasound have the same mechanism of action; the differences between them will be discussed further in Sect. 5.4.

3 Clinical Results

In evaluating the degree of acceleration of bone repair with ultrasound, we base our assessments on statistically established norms for fracture healing. These mean values are derived from clinical experience and from data in the literature. Also, we initially formed control groups of 200 patients for each type of fracture, administering conventional treatment to half the patients in each group and ultrasound treatment to the other half. This provided us with 2 groups of 100 patients each in which the results of conventional and ultrasound therapy could be compared. For less common fracture types, the groups consisted of 50 patients each. In recent years we have ceased to conduct this type of comparison, because our success rates with ultrasound have been so high that the modality has become an established part of our treatment protocol in all cases except those noted previously.

3.1 Radial Fractures

Radial fractures are the most common type of fracture in humans (with Sudeck's dystrophy as the leading complication). Following reduction of the fracture and the application of a dorsal plaster slab, ultrasound treatments are initiated on the 6th day.
- Transducer radiating area: 6.4 cm^2.
- Site of application: over the head of the radius (not covered by plaster).
- Coupling method: direct coupling with oil.
- Insonation technique: dynamic.
- Ultrasound intensity: 0.5 W/cm^2.
- Treatment time: 5 min.
- Number of separate treatments: 10.
- Treatment schedule: daily (except weekends) or on alternate days.

Following standard radiographic views to confirm union, the plaster is removed at 3 weeks (day 21 postfracture). In 86% of patients the fracture site is fully consolidated (radiographically healed). Comparison with average length of immobilization and occupational disability time without ultrasound indicates the following:
- Length of immobilization with ultrasound: 21 days.
- Length of immobilization without ultrasound: 35 days.

- Disability time with ultrasound: 45 days.
- Disability time without ultrasound: 65 days.

The following studies were performed in a group of 50 patients receiving therapeutic ultrasound and in another 50 patients not treated with ultrasound (average age 61.4 years):

- Radiographs on days 7, 21, 35, and 49 postfracture (p.f.).
- Determination of serum alkaline phosphatase, Ca, P, and Zn on days 14, 21, and 35 p.f.
- ^{99m}Tc hydroxylidene diphosphonate scintigraphic studies of both wrists, elbows, and the distal third of the forearm on days 21 and 35 p.f. using a standard anatomic position and imaging technique. Radiotracer uptake was quantified using the ROI (region of interest) method.
- Photon-absorption measurement of the total mineral content of the fracture area on days 21, 28, 35, 49, and 70.
- Measurement of ultrasound absorption at the fracture site on days 21, 35, and 49 using two transducers with a 1.4-cm^2 radiating or receiving area. Transmitting transducer (1.4 cm^2) and receiving transducer (1.4 cm^2) coupled to oscillographs, sound intensity 0.5 W/cm^2.
- Infrared measurement of the skin temperature over the fracture site on days 21, 28, 35, 49, 56, 70, and 84.

These studies, combined with the findings in experimental animals, offer the most compelling proof of the statements made in the introduction. Because the resulting are so convincing, we felt it unnecessary to seek analogous proof for other fracture locations. Comparison of the two patient groups indicated the following:

- Radiographs demonstrate earlier consolidation of fractures treated with ultrasound. Besides the 86% of fractures that were consolidated on day 21, all of the fractures (100%) were radiographically healed by day 35 (Fig. 9). In patients not treated with ultrasound, there was no case in which consolidation was noted on day 21. By day 35, the consolidation rate in these patients was 69% (Fig. 10).
- The following serum alkaline phosphatase levels (Fig. 11) were measured in the patients not treated with ultrasound:
    day 14 p.f.: 2.75 ± 0.62 μmol/l,
    day 21 p.f.: 3.82 ± 0.58 μmol/l,
    day 35 p.f.: 4.38 ± 0.77 μmol/l.

  The following levels were measured in the ultrasound-treated patients:
    day 14 p.f.: 3.72 ± 0.81 μmol/l,
    day 21 p.f.: 4.91 ± 0.78 μmol/l,
    day 35 p.f.: 4.00 ± 0.68 μmol/l.
- Calcium and phosphorus levels showed no changes in either group, while zinc levels showed insignificant borderline changes.

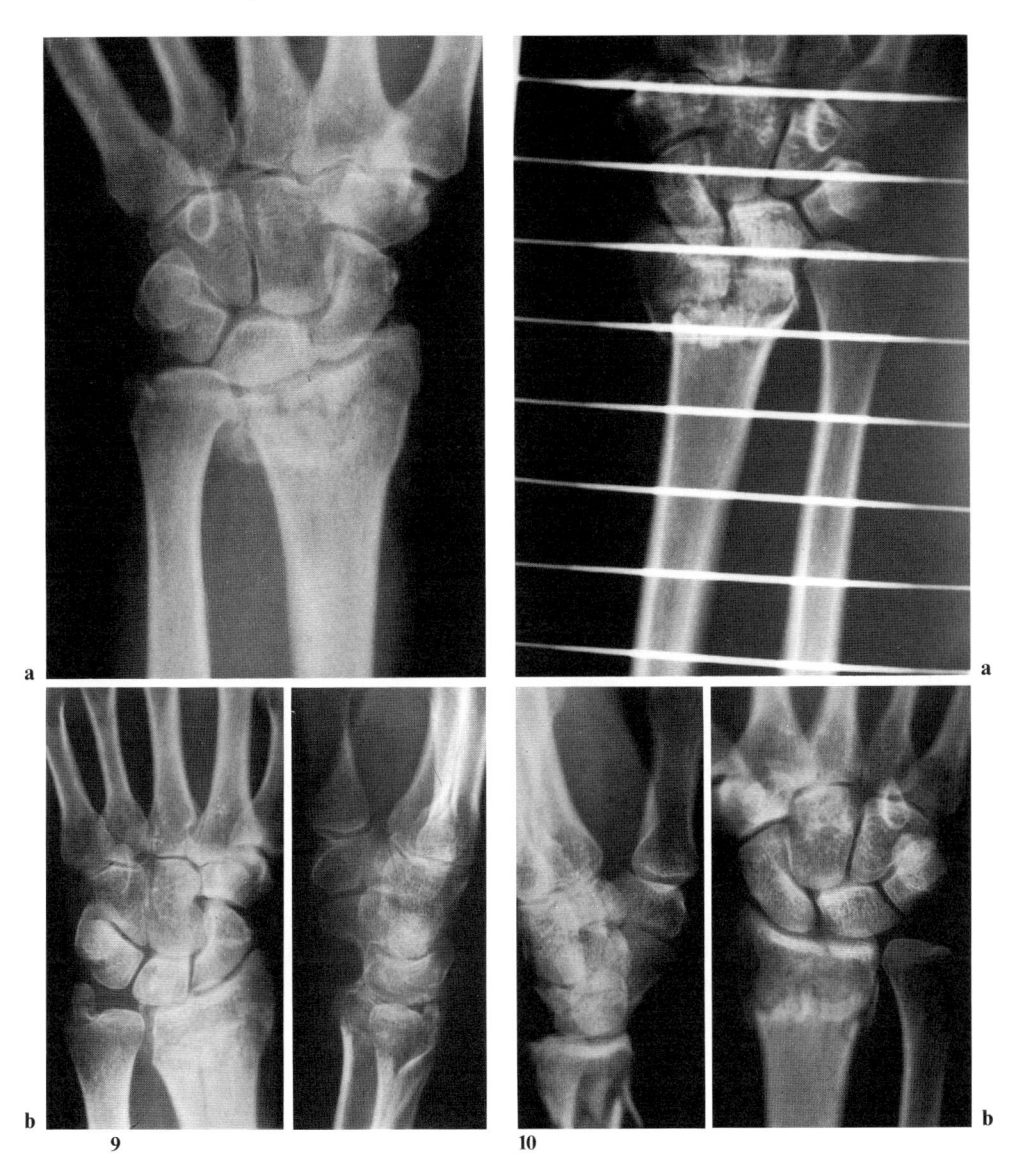

Fig. 9. a Distal radial fracture in a 64-year-old woman. **b** Day 21 p.f., after 10 ultrasound treatments. The fracture is radiographically consolidated

Fig. 10. a Distal radial fracture in a 64-year-old woman. **b** On the 21st day of immobilization, the fracture is not yet consolidated

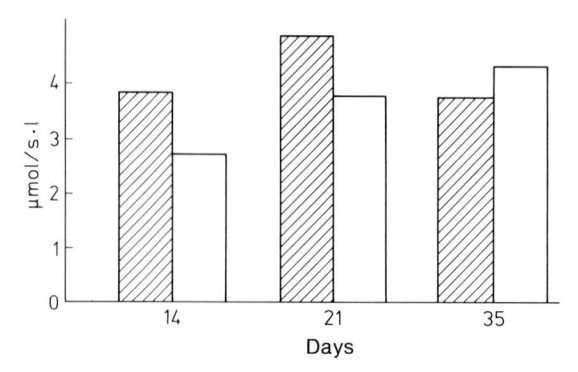

Fig. 11. Serum alkaline phosphatase levels in patients treated with ultrasound (*hatched area*) and patients not treated with ultrasound (*white area*)

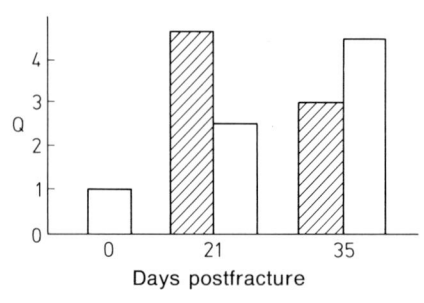

Fig. 12. ROI activity quotient Q in the region of distal radial fractures treated with ultrasound (*hatched area*) and without ultrasound (*white area*)

- The scintigraphic ROI activity quotients Q (Fig. 12) in patients not treated with ultrasound were as follows:
    day 21 p.f.: 2.41, $\sigma_n - 1 = \pm 0.52$;
    day 35 p.f.: 4.32, $\sigma_n - 1 = \pm 0.64$ ($\sigma_n - 1$; standard deviation for test).
  The activity quotients in the 27 ultrasound-treated patients were as follows:
    day 21 p.f.: 4.65, $\sigma_n - 1 = \pm 0.66$;
    day 35 p.f.: 3.07, $\sigma_n - 1 = \pm 0.69$.
- Total mineral analysis of the fracture area in patients not treated with ultrasound indicated:
    on day 21 66%,
    on day 28 74%,
    on day 35 81%,
    on day 49 91%,
    on day 70 100%
  of the value in the contralateral uninjured radius.

Table 1. Ultrasound treatment and skin temperature: temperature increase (in °C) over the fracture site relative to the uninjured side

Days postfracture	Without ultrasound	With ultrasound
21	+ 1.6	+ 2.4
28	+ 2.0	+ 1.6
35	+ 1.6	+ 0.9
42	+ 2.35	+ 0.5
49	+ 1.4	0.0
56	+ 1.1	0.0
70	+ 0.7	0.0
84	0.0	0.0

Analysis following ultrasound stimulation indicated a bone index:
 on day 21 of 109%,
 on day 28 of 167%,
 on day 49 of 150%,
 on day 70 of 131%
relative to the contralateral unfractured radius.

- The ultrasound absorption measurements are of particular interest in terms of the rate of fracture healing. The following values were measured for the percentage of the transmitted ultrasound intensity that was absorbed at the fracture site:
 Without ultrasound treatment:
  day 21 p.f.: 37% ± 9%,
  day 35 p.f.: 53% ± 13%.
 Following ultrasound treatment:
  day 21 p.f.: 53% ± 10%,
  day 35 p.f.: 74% ± 11%.
- Skin temperatures were measured with the Pyrovar infrared thermometer over the fracture site and over the contralateral distal, uninjured forearm. As the data in Table 1 indicate, the rate of normalization was significantly more rapid in the patients who received therapeutic ultrasound.

The foregoing studies clearly demonstrate that the course of fracture healing and the return to functional soundness are accelerated under the influence of ultrasonic energy.

3.2 Scaphoid Fractures

Without going into the classification of these fractures, and disregarding the very rare displaced fractures and fractures requiring primary operation, it will be noted that the essential problem with scaphoid fractures is the need for prolonged immobilization (6–15 weeks or more depending on the type of fracture) and the high rate of nonunion (2%–5% of all cases). Initial treatment consists of immobilizing the fracture in a long arm cast or short arm cast; we prefer the latter.

Starting on day 6, ultrasound is administered through a cast window 2×3 cm in size over the scaphoid bone. This does not compromise the stability of the cast. Technique: oil coupling of small transducer (radiating area $1.4\,\text{cm}^2$) moved in a circular pattern. Ultrasound intensity $0.1-0.3\,\text{W/cm}^2$, treatment time 5 min every other day, total of 15–20 treatments.

After 6 weeks' immobilization with ultrasound treatments, 91% of all fractures are radiographically healed. Another 8% heal with an additional 2 weeks' immobilization and ultrasound therapy (Fig. 13).

Comparison with a control group indicated the following average lengths of immobilization and disability:
- Immobilization with ultrasound: 45 days.
- Immobilization without ultrasound: 90 days.
- Disability time with ultrasound: 75 days.
- Disability time without ultrasound: 120 days.

The same studies were performed in our patients with scaphoid fractures as in those with radial fractures (see Sect. 3.1). The results are similar, so they will not be presented in detail. To summarize, it may be said that ultrasound stimulation can significantly shorten the duration of treatment and immobilization, prevent the development of nonunion, and minimize the need for operative treatment (Fig. 14).

In two patients fracture healing was not achieved, and it became necessary to proceed with operative treatment.

3.3 Metacarpal Fractures (Fig. 15)

Following reduction and fixation (closed or open), ultrasound treatments are started on the 6th day. If the fracture has been functionally stabilized by rigid internal fixation or immobilized in a waterproof cast, water immersion treatment (using low- or high-frequency ultrasound) is recommended as it offers the advantage of absolute "coupling." With high-frequency ultrasound, an intensity of $0.3\,\text{W/cm}^2$ is used. With an ordinary cast, ultrasound is administered at $0.1\,\text{W/cm}^2$ through a window over the fracture site using the small transducer. If windowing of the cast is too difficult, ultrasound stimulation can be applied indirectly through the corresponding finger or forearm bone, using an intensity of $0.4-0.6\,\text{W/cm}^2$. Regardless of the site or mode of application, a total of 10–12 treatments are given on alternate days, each lasting 3 min.

Comparison with a control group indicated the following:
- Immobilization with ultrasound: 31 days.
- Immobilization without ultrasound: 46 days.
- Disability time with ultrasound: 48 days.
- Disability time without ultrasound: 62 days.

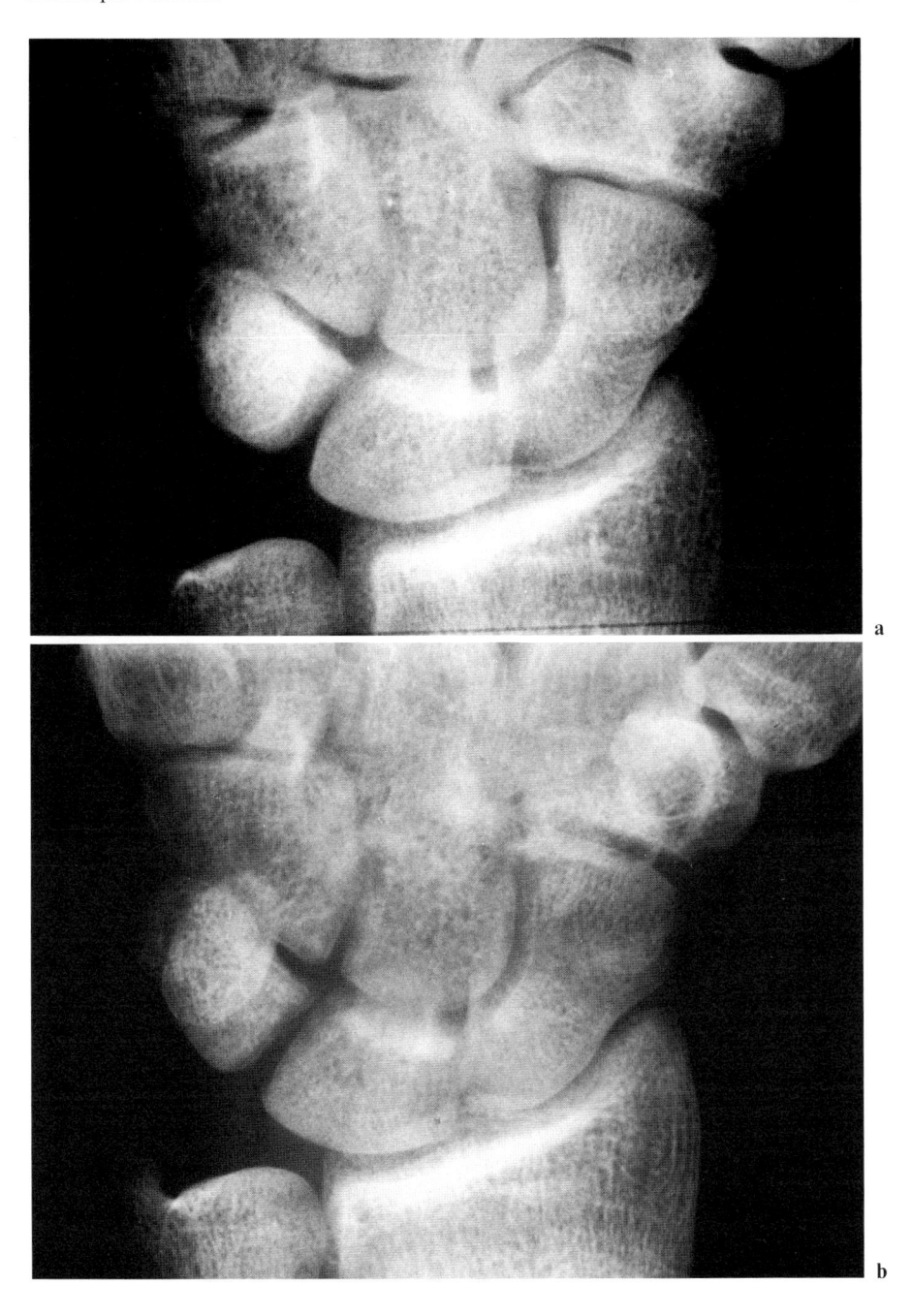

Fig. 13. a Scaphoid fracture in a 31-year-old man. **b** Day 45 p.f., after 16 ultrasound treatments. The fracture is healed

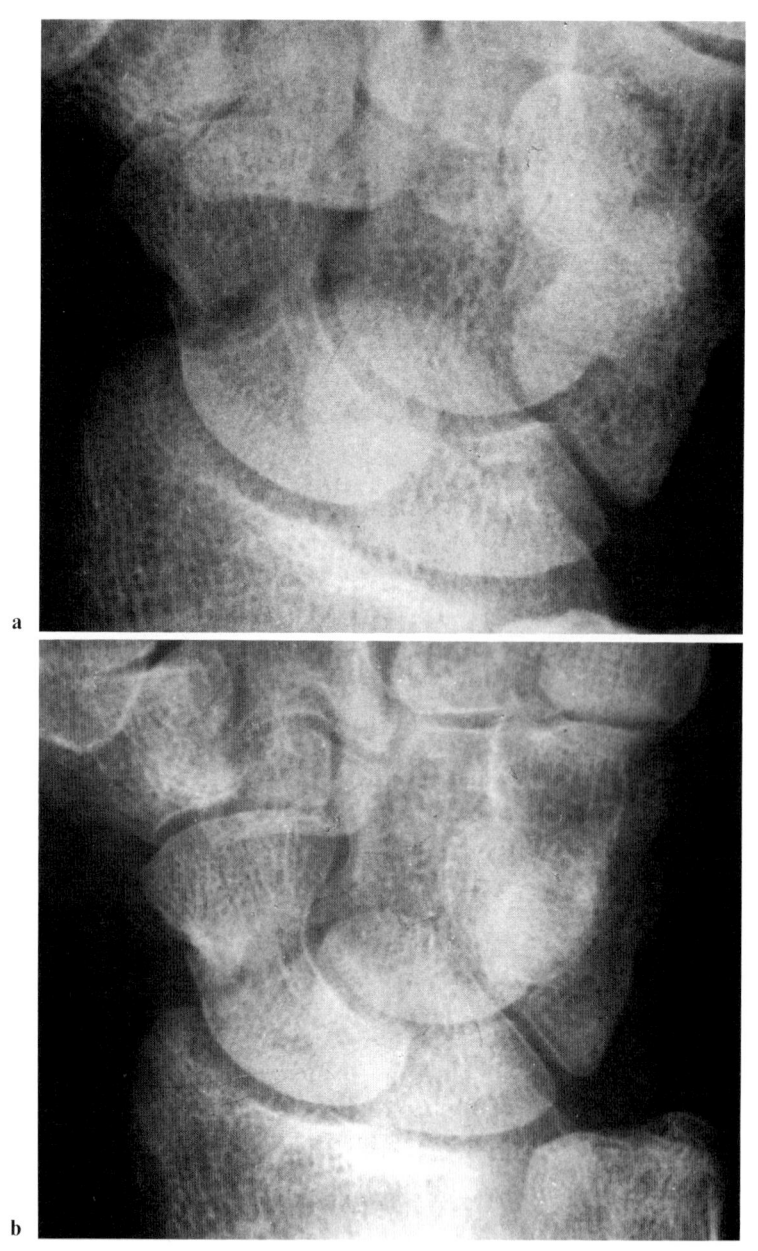

Fig. 14. a Scaphoid fracture in a 52-year-old woman who presented 6 weeks after the injury with delayed callus formation and impending nonunion. **b** Day 56 after immobilization and 20 ultrasound treatments. The fracture is consolidated

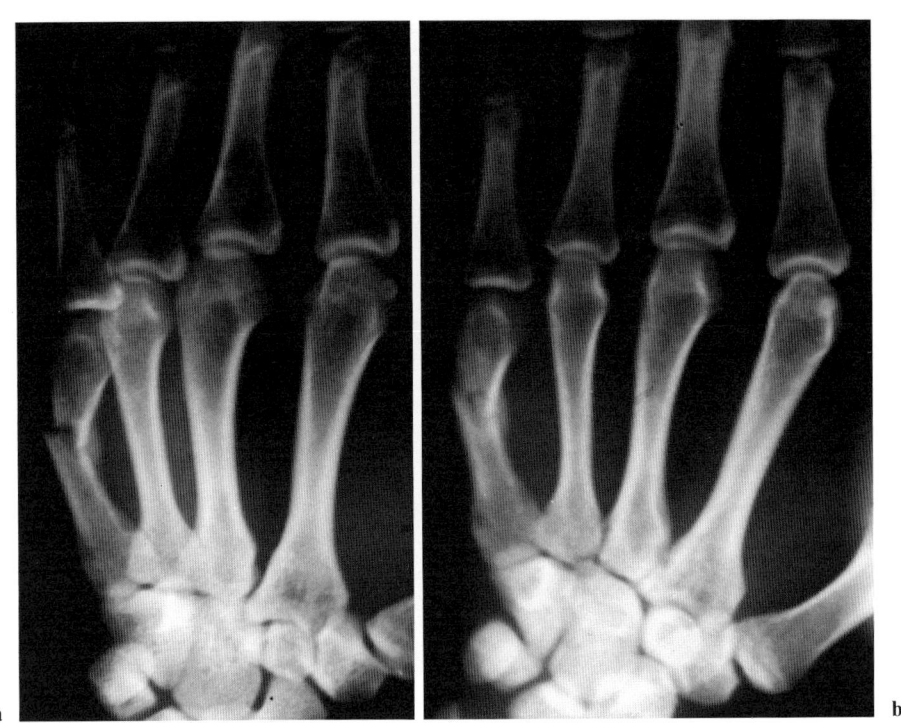

Fig. 15. a Metacarpal fracture in a 37-year-old man. **b** Day 30 p.f., after 10 ultrasound treatments. The fracture is healed

3.4 Phalangeal Fractures (Fig. 16)

Ultrasound therapy is started on the 6th day following closed or open reduction and immobilization of the injury. Water immersion is the recommended mode of treatment (see Sect. 3.3). Alternatively, the ultrasound may be transmitted through the metacarpal ray of the fractured phalanx. The intensity is 0.3 W/cm^2 for water immersion and 0.5 W/cm^2 for metacarpal insonation. A total of 8 treatments, each lasting 3 min, are administered on alternate days.

Comparison with a control group indicated the following:
- Immobilization with ultrasound: 28 days.
- Immobilization without ultrasound: 42 days.

Length of disability is essentially the same for both groups due to the influence of occupation, age (some children), and concomitant injuries.

3.5 Forearm Fractures (Figs. 17 and 18)

Ultrasound treatments are started on the 6th day after closed or open reduction, insonating through a cast window over the fracture or fractures. The

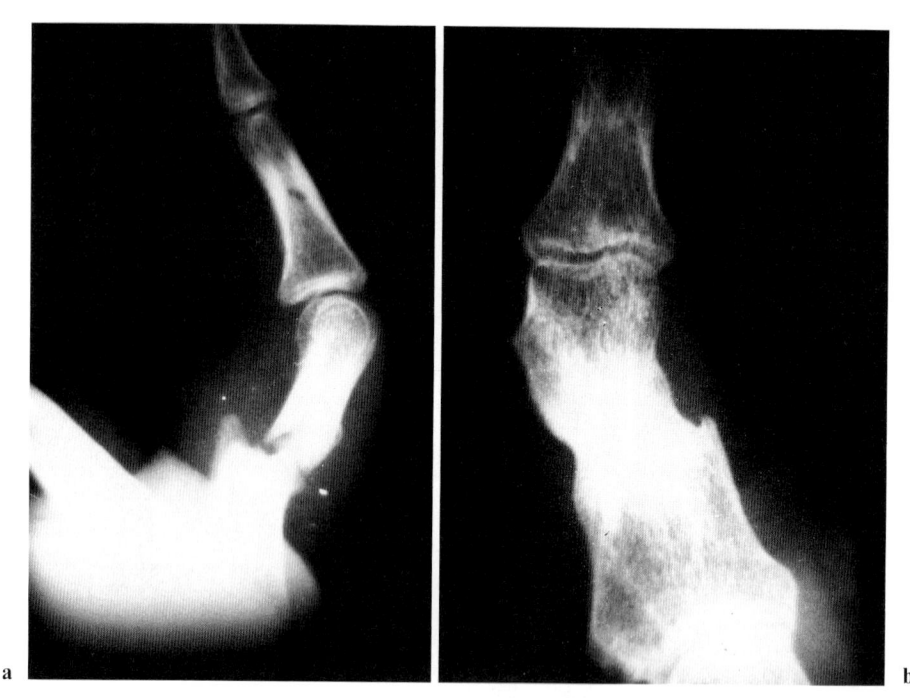

Fig. 16. a Fracture of the proximal phalanx of the index finger in a 28-year-old male. **b** Day 30 p.f., after 12 ultrasound treatments. The fracture is healed

window may be placed over the fracture site or over the olecranon. The small transducer is oil-coupled to the skin using circular motions and an intensity of 0.3 W/cm². A total of 10–12 treatments, each lasting 3 min, are given on alternate days.

Comparison with a control group indicated the following:
– Immobilization with ultrasound: 39 days.
– Immobilization without ultrasound: 60 days.
– Disability time with ultrasound: 52 days.
– Disability time without ultrasound: 86 days.

With a conservatively or operatively treated fracture of the olecranon (Figs. 19 and 20), ultrasound treatments are started on the 6th day through a cast window using an intensity of 0.1 W/cm². For indirect stimulation, the styloid process of the ulna can be insonated at 0.5 W/cm² (10–12 treatments on alternate days). The average time to complete union is 3 weeks.

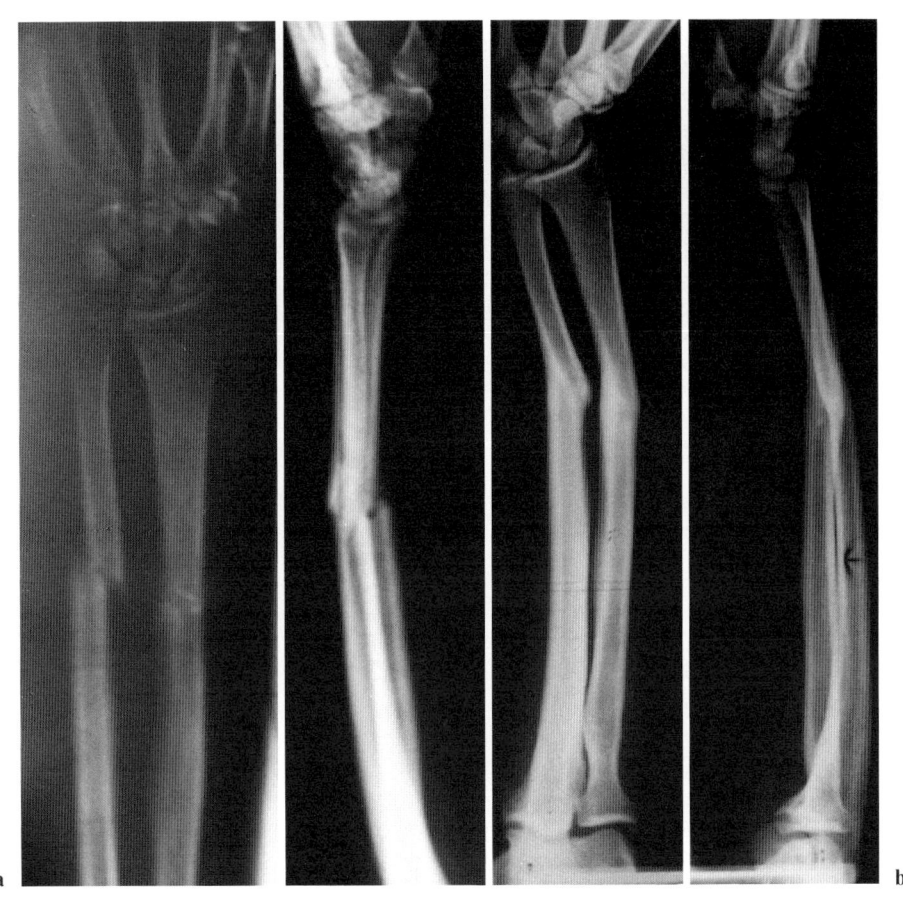

Fig. 17. a Fracture of both forearm bones in a 21-year-old male who declined operative treatment. The fractures were immobilized in plaster. **b** Day 42 p.f., after 12 ultrasound treatments. The fractures are healed with slight angular deformity

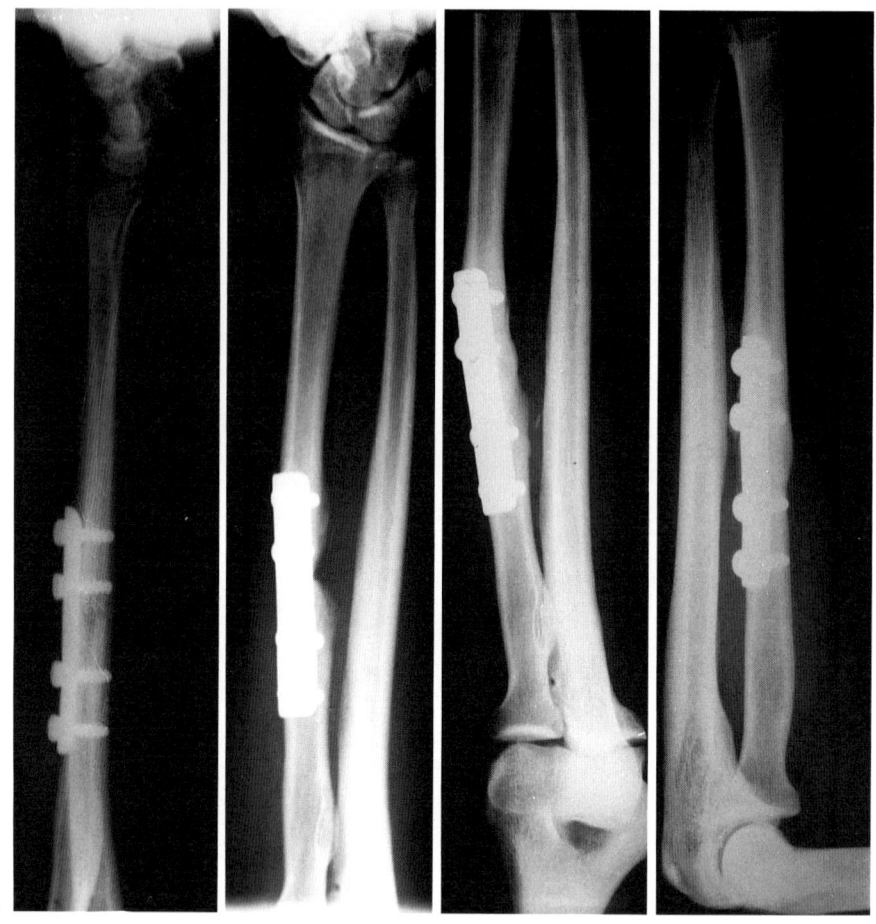

Fig. 18. a Fracture of the radial shaft in a 43-year-old female, managed by internal fixation due to a bone defect. Ultrasound treatments were started on the 6th postoperative day. **b** Day 26, after 12 ultrasound treatments. The defect is bridged, and the fracture is healed

Fig. 19. a Displaced olecranon fracture in a 43-year-old male, stabilized by tension-band fixation on the day of the injury. **b** Day 21 p.f., after 12 ultrasound treatments. The fracture is healed with good function

Fig. 20. a Minimally displaced olecranon fracture (82-year-old female). Because of the patient's age, the fracture was immobilized with a splint. **b** Day 22, after 12 ultrasound treatments. The fracture is solid, and function is good

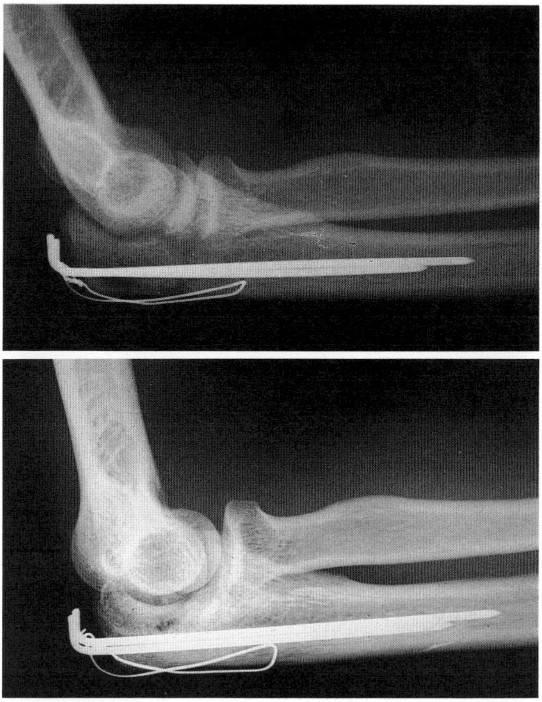

a

19 b

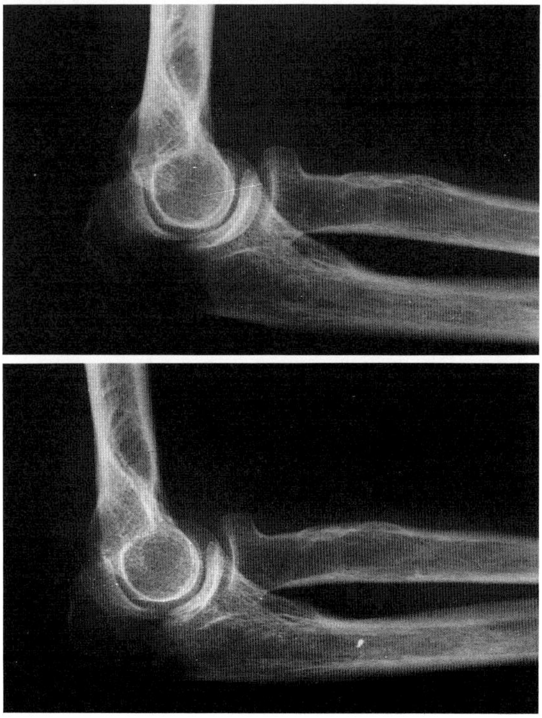

a

20 b

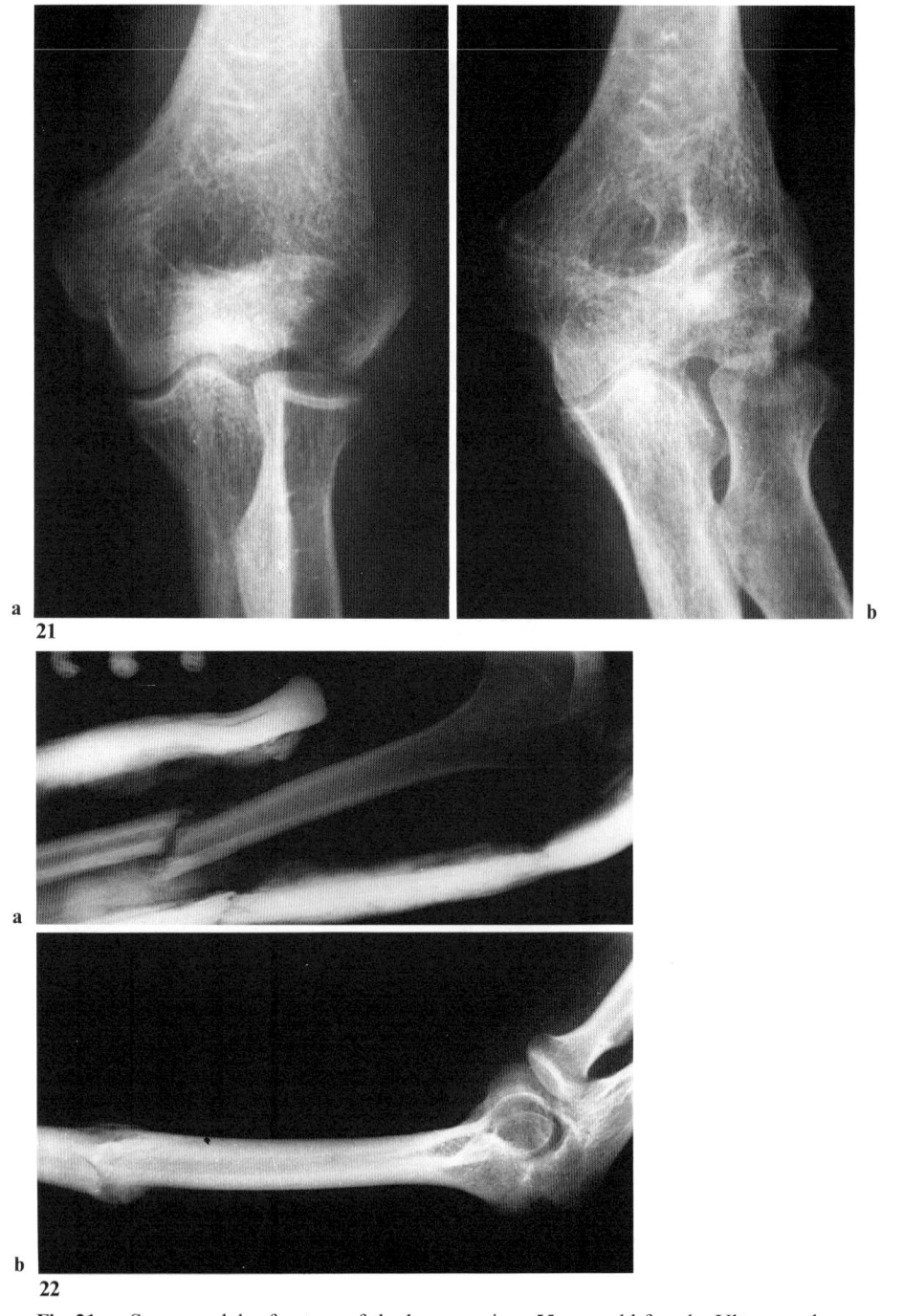

Fig. 21. a Supracondylar fracture of the humerus in a 55-year-old female. Ultrasound was applied directly through a window in the long arm cast. **b** Day 25, after 12 treatments. The fracture is functionally stable

Fig. 22. a Humeral shaft fracture in a 38-year-old male who declined operative treatment. Fracture was stabilized with an abduction splint and directly insonated through a window in the cast. **b** Day 35, after 15 ultrasound treatments. The fracture is consolidated

3.6 Humeral Fractures

Ultrasound therapy is started on the 6th day regardless of whether closed or open reduction is used. With condylar and supracondylar fractures (Fig. 21), ultrasound is applied through a cast window directly over the fracture site using a small transducer, oil-coupled, operated at an intensity of $0.1-0.2$ W/cm^2. A total of 10–12 treatments are given, each lasting 3 min. Total fracture treatment time can generally be shortened by 40% with this regimen.

With a fracture of the humeral shaft (Fig. 22), ultrasound is applied either through a cast window using an intensity of $0.2-0.3$ W/cm^2 or from the epicondyles at an intensity of 0.5 W/cm^2. A total of 2 to 15 treatments, each lasting 3–5 min, are administered on alternate days. Total treatment time is shortened by 35%.

Subcapital humeral fractures (Fig. 23) are insonated directly at 0.2 W/cm^2 or from the epicondyles at 0.5 W/cm^2, with 10–12 treatments given on alternate days. Treatment time is shortened by 40%. (The very wide age range, the large percentage of elderly patients, the diversity of fracture sites, and the varying problems of immobilization are significant factors in the management of humeral fractures. Therefore data on healing time reduction are expressed in percent.)

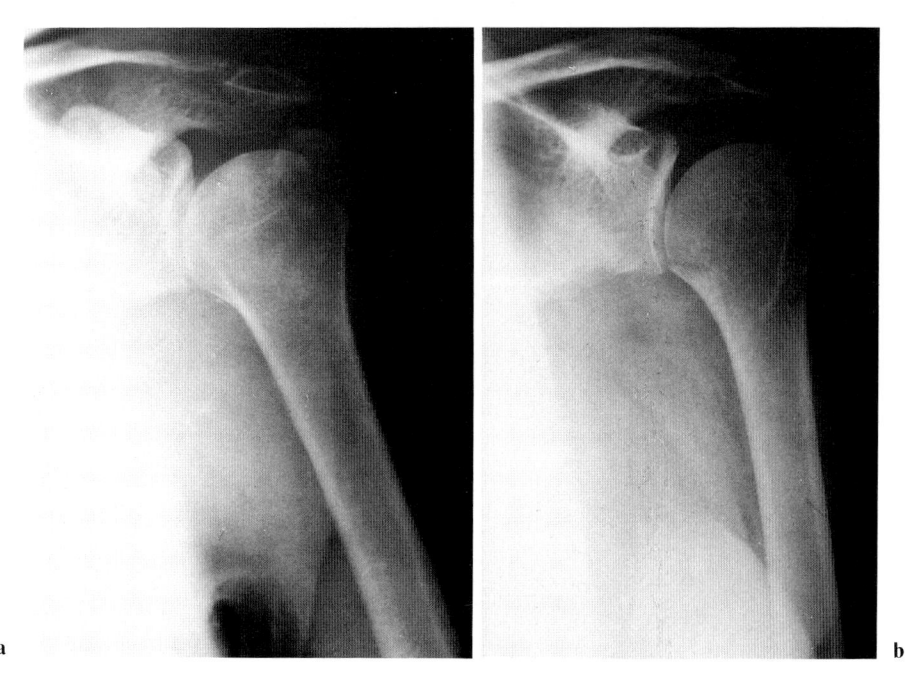

Fig. 23. a Subcapital fracture of the humerus with avulsion of the greater tuberosity in a 54-year-old female. **b** Day 24, after 12 ultrasound treatments. The fracture is functionally stable, the arm functionally sound

3.7 Clavicular Fractures (Fig. 24)

These fractures are usually immobilized with a figure-of-eight bandage. In cases managed conservatively as well as prior to operation, ultrasound treatments are started on the 6th day. Ultrasound is applied directly over the fracture site with the small transducer at $0.1-0.2$ W/cm^2. A total of 6 treatments, each lasting 3 min, are administered on alternate days.
- Immobilization with ultrasound: 20 days.
- Immobilization without ultrasound: 35 days.
- Disability time with ultrasound: 25 days.
- Disability time without ultrasound: 35 days.

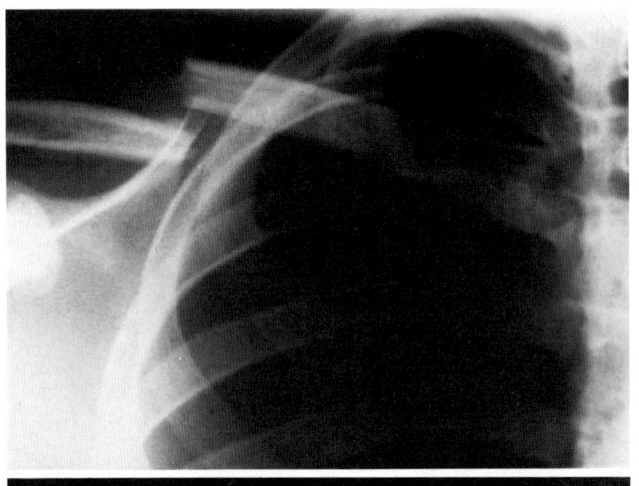

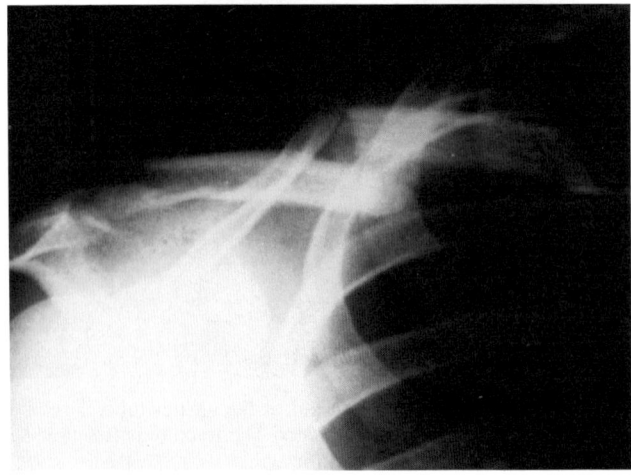

Fig. 24. a Midshaft fracture of the clavicle in a 24-year-old male, managed by closed reduction and a figure-of-eight bandage. **b** Day 19, after 10 ultrasound treatments. The fracture is solid

3.8 Malleolar Fractures (Figs. 25–27)

In this very diverse patient group, ultrasound treatments are started on the 6th day in cases managed by closed or open reduction. The fracture site can be insonated directly with a small transducer operated at 0.2–0.3 W/cm^2. Unilateral fractures are given a total of 10–14 treatments on alternate days; bilateral fractures are treated daily, insonating the medial side one day and the lateral side the next.

In cases managed operatively or immobilized in a waterproof cast (with a large window), the optimum mode of ultrasound treatment is water immersion using a low-frequency therapy unit. This is advantageous in terms of improving tissue oxygen supply and promoting blood flow – effects that are particularly beneficial in fracture-dislocations. A total of 15–20 treatments, each lasting 5 min, are given on alternate days.

Average results in nondislocated malleolar fractures:
- Immobilization with ultrasound: 40 days.
- Immobilization without ultrasound: 70 days.
- Disability time with ultrasound: 70 days.
- Disability time without ultrasound: 140 days.

Average results in fracture-dislocations:
- Immobilization with ultrasound: 60 days.
- Immobilization without ultrasound: 95 days.
- Disability time with ultrasound: 92 days.
- Disability time without ultrasound: 155 days.

3.9 Tibial Fractures (Figs. 28 and 29)

Like malleolar fractures, these fractures are quite diverse with respect to type, location, and management by open or closed reduction, and only average values can be stated. Ultrasound therapy is started 1 week after closed or open reduction and may be administered directly over the fracture site on the upper tibia or indirectly from the malleolar area. An intensity of 0.2–0.3 W/cm^2 is used directly over the fracture, 0.2 W/cm^2 for insonating the proximal tibia when a Küntscher nail is in place, 0.5–0.6 W/cm^2 when a Küntscher nail is not used, and 0.3–0.5 W/cm^2 for insonating over the malleoli. A total of 14–20 treatments, each of 3 min duration, are given on alternate days.

Average results:
- Immobilization with ultrasound: 84 days.
- Immobilization without ultrasound: 120 days.
- Disability time with ultrasound: 110 days.
- Disability time without ultrasound: 159 days.

26   Clinical Results

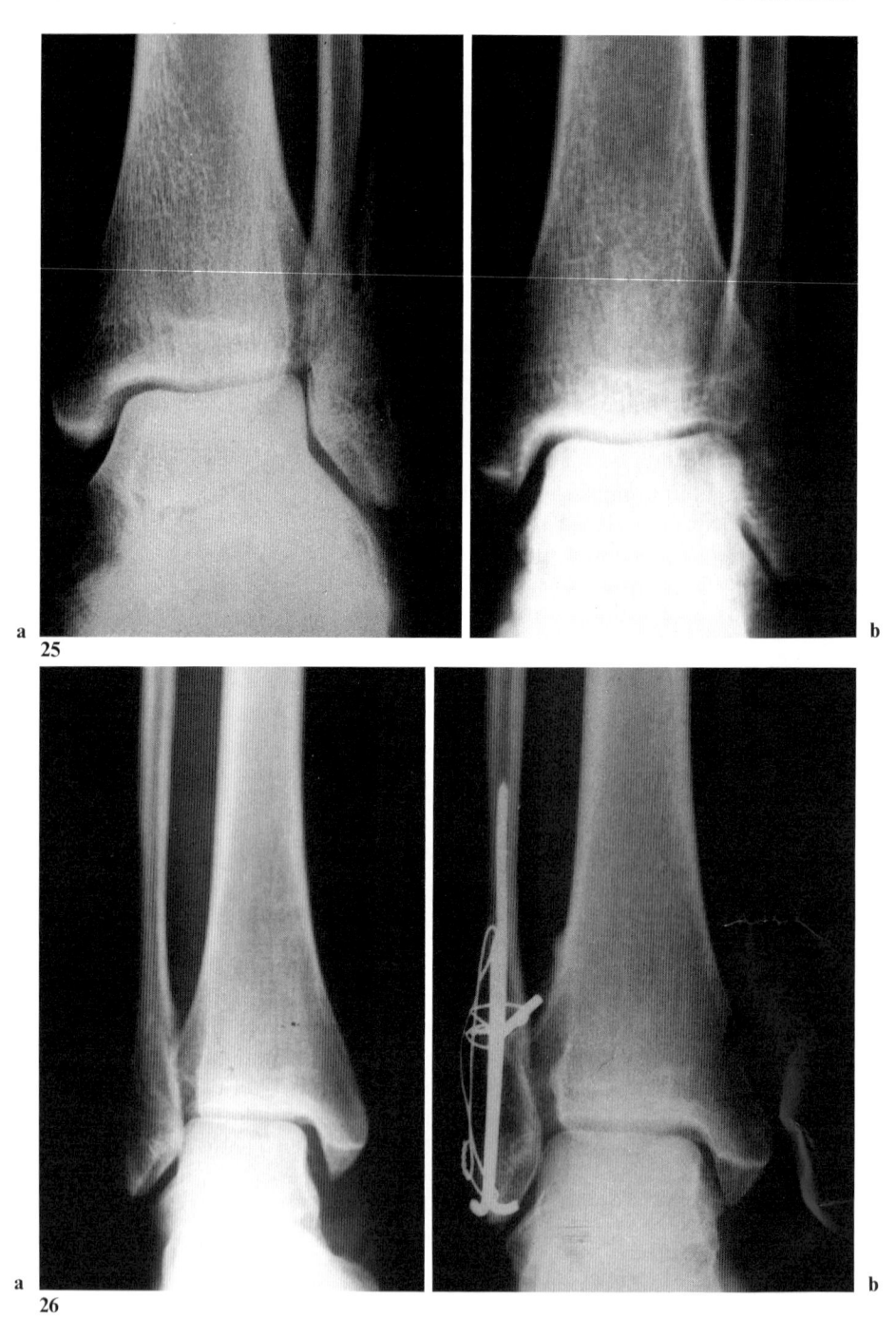

a   b
25

a   b
26

Tibial Fractures

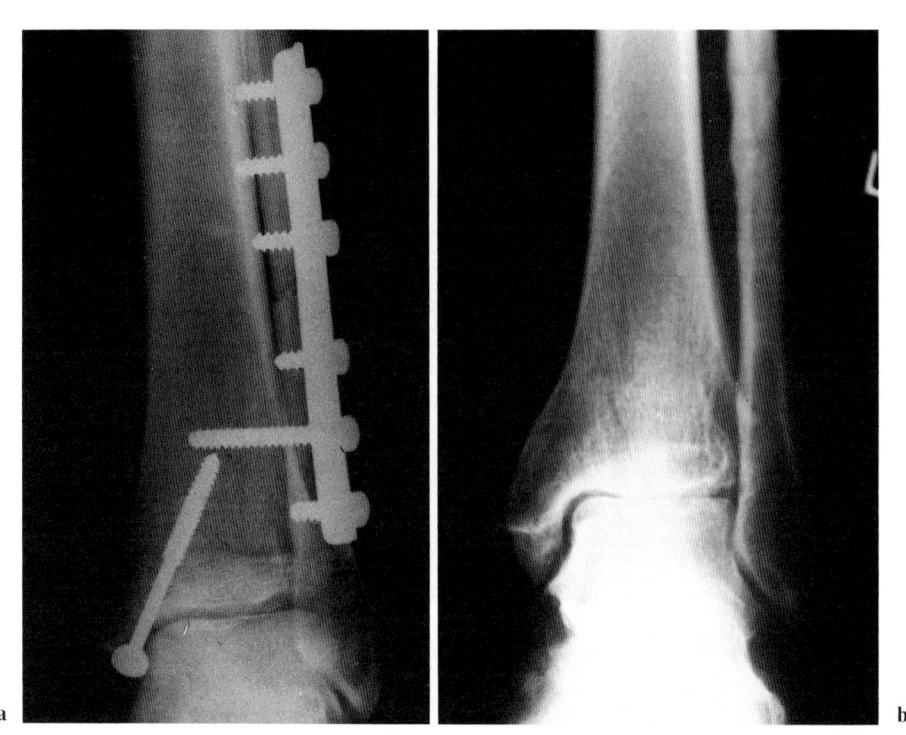

Fig. 27. a Bimalleolar fracture-dislocation (25-year-old female), managed by immediate operation and 20 ultrasound treatments. On day 60 p.f. the fractures are healed. **b** Appearance after removal of the internal fixation material illustrates the good acoustic conductivity of the metal. The bone structure is preserved

Fig. 25. a Lateral malleolar fracture in a 19-year-old female. **b** Day 40 p.f., after 14 treatments. The fracture is healed with good function

Fig. 26. a Weber Type C malleolar fracture in a 44-year-old female, managed by operation and subsequent ultrasound treatments. **b** On day 50 p.f., following internal fixation and 14 treatments. Normal weight bearing

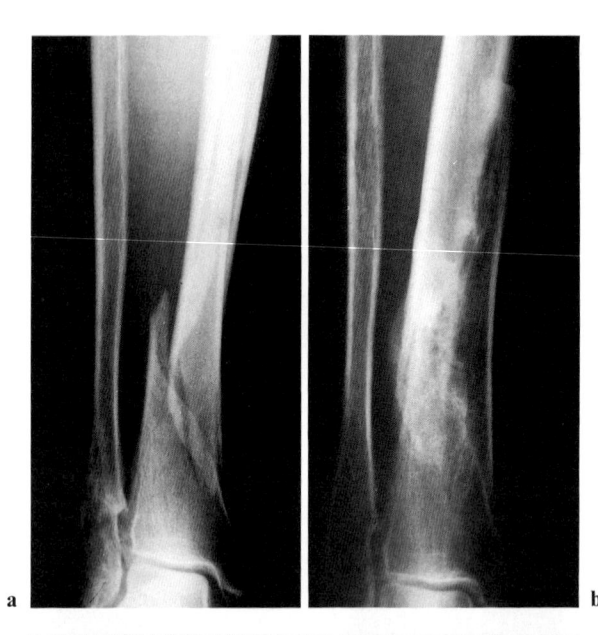

Fig. 28. a Torsional fracture of the distal third of the tibia (55-year-old male) managed by closed reduction and immobilization in a long leg cast. Fracture was directly insonated through a cast window. **b** Day 58 p.f., after 18 ultrasound treatments. The fracture can bear weight normally

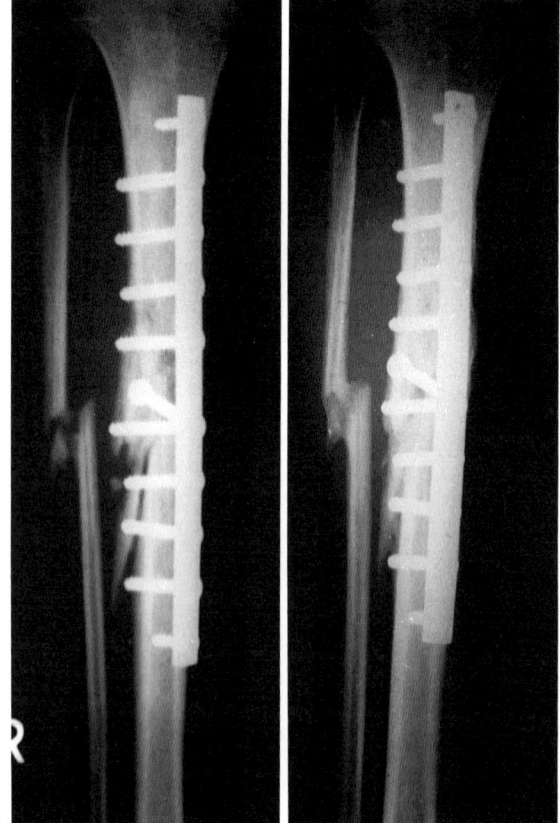

Fig. 29. a Comminuted midshaft tibial fracture (48-year-old female) managed by immediate internal fixation. **b** Day 35 p.f., after 15 insonations. The fracture is stable on weight bearing

3.10 Femoral Fractures (Fig. 30)

In operatively or conservatively managed avulsion fractures of the femoral condyles, the condyles are directly insonated starting on day 6 using an intensity of $0.2-0.3$ W/cm^2. A total of 10–14 treatments are given. Since most diaphyseal fractures are managed operatively, ultrasound treatments are started 1 week after operation. The fracture site may be insonated directly at 0.5 W/cm^2, or ultrasound may be applied over the greater trochanter at 0.6 W/cm^2 or through the condyles at 0.5 W/cm^2. A total of 12–20 treatments lasting 3–5 min are administered on alternate days.

Average results:
- Immobilization with ultrasound: 75 days.
- Immobilization without ultrasound: 120 days.
- Disability time with ultrasound: 90 days.
- Disability time without ultrasound: 120 days.

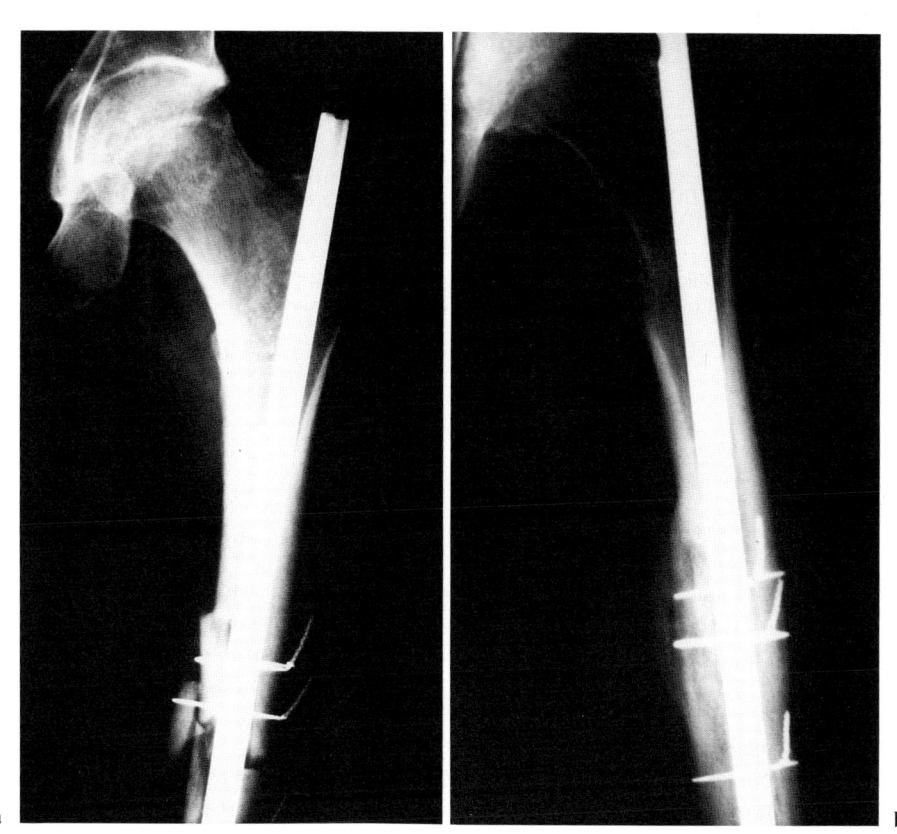

Fig. 30. a Comminuted middle-third fracture of the femur (34-year-old male) stabilized with a Küntscher nail cerclage wires. Ultrasound was administered through the proximal fragment. **b** Day 67 p.f., after 18 ultrasound treatments. The fracture is able to bear weight

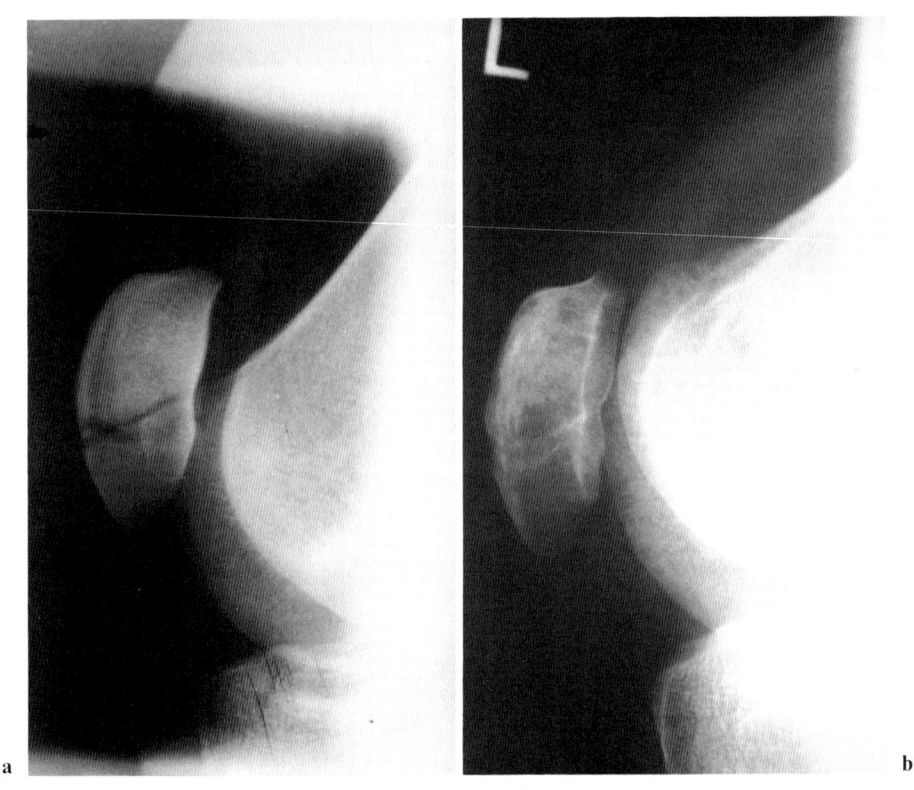

Fig. 31. a Nondisplaced patellar fracture (52-year-old female), managed by immobilization. **b** Day 24, after 12 ultrasound treatments. The fracture is functionally stable

3.11 Patellar Fractures (Fig. 31)

Ultrasound is started on the 6th day after operative or conservative treatment. The fracture is insonated directly through a windowed cast at $0.1-0.2$ W/cm^2 using the small transducer. A total of $8-10$ treatments are given on alternate days.

Average results:
- Immobilization with ultrasound (operative treatment): 21 days.
  Immobilization without ultrasound (nonoperative treatment): 30 days.
- Immobilization without ultrasound: 45 days.
- Disability time with ultrasound: 68 days.
- Disability time without ultrasound: 90 days.

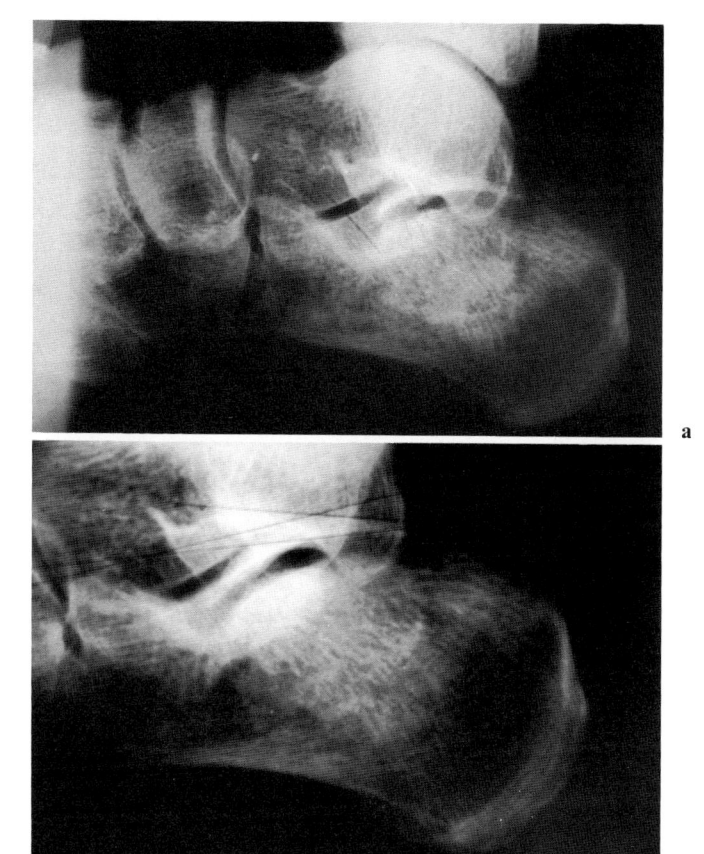

Fig. 32. a Nondisplaced calcaneal fracture (53-year-old male), immobilized in a plaster cast with a large window. **b** Day 40 p.f. after 16 ultrasound treatments. The fracture is able to bear weight

3.12 Calcaneal Fractures (Fig. 32)

One week after closed reduction, the fracture is insonated through a windowed cast at 0.3 W/cm^2 using the small transducer. A total of 15–20 treatments of 5 min duration are given on alternate days. The window can be placed lateral or medial to the bone or directly over the heel.

With a waterproof cast, we recommend 5-min water immersion treatments using low-frequency ultrasound. This offers the advantages of better acoustic coupling and improved blood flow.

Average results:
- Immobilization with ultrasound: 65 days.
- Immobilization without ultrasound: 90 days.
- Disability time with ultrasound: 100 days.
- Disability time without ultrasound: 125 days.

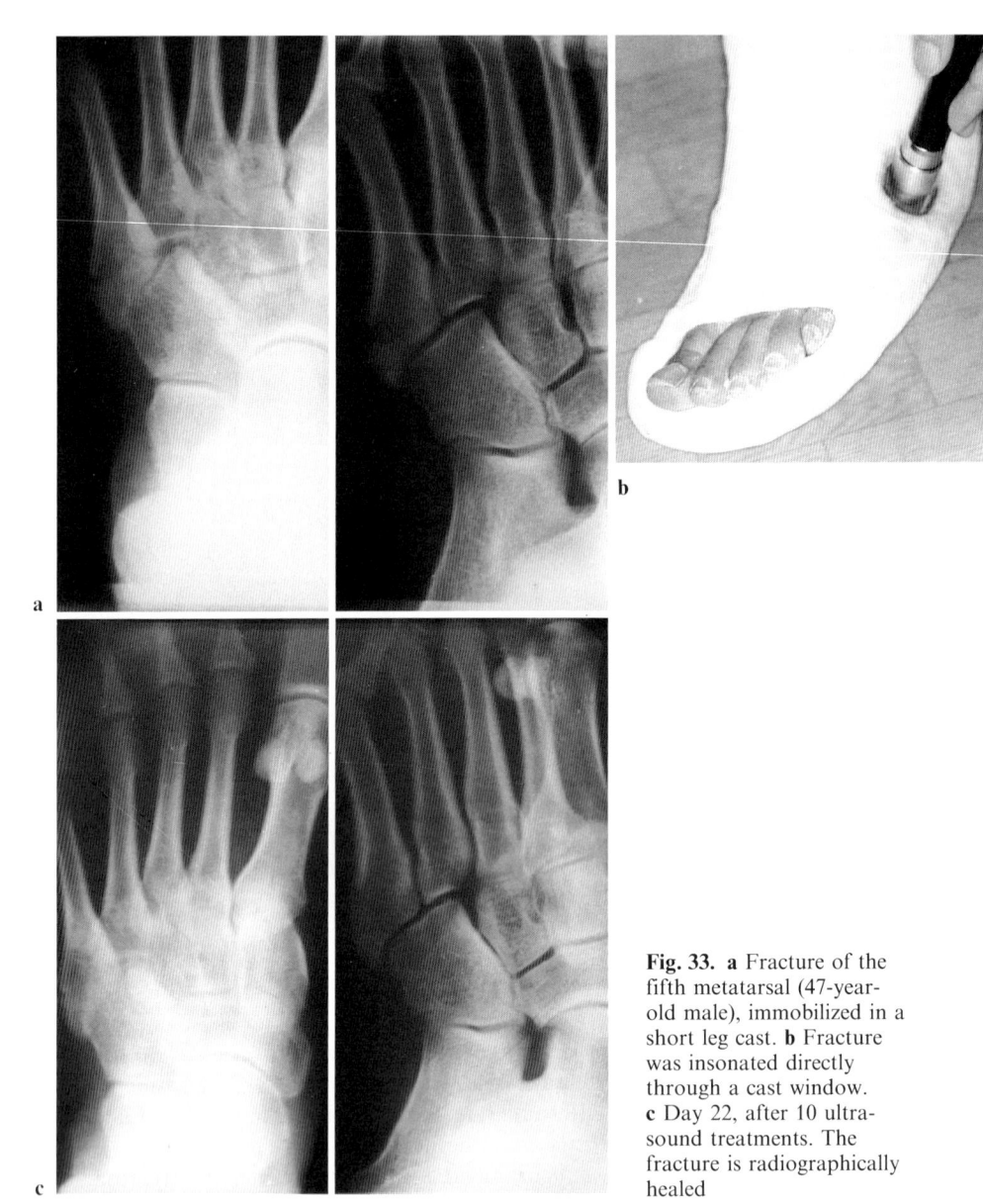

Fig. 33. a Fracture of the fifth metatarsal (47-year-old male), immobilized in a short leg cast. **b** Fracture was insonated directly through a cast window. **c** Day 22, after 10 ultrasound treatments. The fracture is radiographically healed

3.13 Metatarsal Fractures (Fig. 33)

Treatments are started 6 days after the fracture or operation, insonating through a window directly over the fracture with a small transducer operated at 0.2–0.3 W/cm^2. A total of 10–12, 3-min treatments are given on alternate days. If the cast is difficult to window over the fracture, the ultrasound can be applied through a window over the calcaneus or to the large toe using an intensity of 0.5–0.6 W/cm^2.

We also recommend low-frequency insonation in a water bath, giving a total of 12–15 treatments of 5 min duration on alternate days. In patients with associated soft-tissue injuries or ulcerations, low-frequency ultrasound is particularly beneficial for promoting blood flow.

Average results:
- Immobilization with ultrasound: 25 days.
- Immobilization without ultrasound: 45 days.
- Disability time with ultrasound: 65 days.
- Disability time without ultrasound: 85 days.

4 How did we Come to use Ultrasound?

In the search for a way to stimulate bone repair, and after futile attempts to shorten the healing process by pharmacologic and hormonal methods, our attention turned to a method successfully used in technology (especially structural engineering) whereby vibrations are used to affect the density of solids and other media. A review of the literature shows that at least 46 different approaches have been taken in an attempt to stimulate bone repair, including operative procedures, chemical and biochemical agents, drug treatments, and physical methods. Operative procedures have proven effective in suitably selected cases. Of the physical methods, efficacy has been demonstrated for electrical stimulation and ultrasonic therapy. The basic mechanism of action of both modalities is the piezoelectric effect. But treatment with ultrasound offers several advantages over electrical stimulation: (1) the instruments can be used for various applications, (2) the necessary equipment is widely available, (3) ultrasound therapy causes no side effects or complications, and (4) therapeutic ultrasound has been used clinically for 30 years. It was a natural step to apply the compaction properties of ultrasonic energy familiar in engineering to the compaction of callus tissue at a fracture site. This line of reasoning led us to consider the use of vibrational energy in the broadest sense.

In experiments on rabbits in which one tibia was osteotomized and immobilized by internal fixation, we investigated the effects of low-frequency vibrations and later of high-frequency vibrations on the callus tissue from a clinical, radiographic, and histologic standpoint. Low-frequency stimulation was produced manually and also with a low-frequency generator, while high-frequency vibrations were produced with an ultrasound machine.

The treatments were started 1 week postoperatively. This was felt to allow ample time for organization of the fracture hematoma, which in rabbits is complete by the 3rd day, and also for the fibrous phase of the healing process.

The main goal of the experiments was stimulation of the primary callus. To ensure an optimum treatment regimen, special preliminary experiments were done to define the timing, dose level, and duration of treatments. The following protocol was devised: Treatments of 2 min duration were started 1 week postoperatively and repeated on alternate days until a total of 4 treatments had been given. Then, in the 2nd postoperative week, the animals were clinically and radiographically examined. They were sacrificed at the end of the 3rd week, and the operated extremities were removed and stored in formalin solution.

For the preparation of histologic specimens, the fracture site was excised with wide margins using a small power saw. The specimen was fixed in ordinary formalin (1:4), and 5-mm-thick slices were cut and carefully decalcified in Komplexen III (corresponds to Titriplex Merck). Survey sections were prepared with the MSR microtome. The sections were then stained with hematoxylin-eosin and von Kossa's stain.

A second group of animals that underwent osteotomy and internal fixation but received no stimulatory treatments served as controls. At 3 weeks the fractures in this group were neither clinically nor radiographically solid. Histologically, the organization of the fracture hematoma is complete by that time, and there is maximum mobilization of mesenchymal tissue. In some cases there is a transition to primary callus with its fibrous, cartilaginous, and capillary elements. The major stimulus for callus formation is from the periosteum.

Another group of animals was treated by manual vibration (intermittent vibratory massage with the tips of two fingers, directed at right angles to the limb axis). The frequency was 180–200 strokes/min. It was found that this type of massage had no clinically, radiographically, or histologically demonstrable stimulatory effect on callus formation. Neither was the time course of callus formation delayed in relation to the control group.

In the machine experiments on the effect of low-frequency stimulation on callus tissue, the vibrations were produced by a low-frequency generator (RC generator) whose output was connected to a power amplifier. The amplifier was able to make necessary frequency adjustments and impart vibratory motion to a plate, which shook the limb. Frequency and acceleration were monitored with the KD 1 accelerometer (Metra-Radebeul Co.) and an oscillograph. With the apparatus described, vibrations up to 20 kHz could be produced under the same conditions. One matter of interest in this investigation was whether the mechanism of action of the vibrations was based on acceleration (the speed of the motion) or amplitude (the path length of the motion).

Low frequencies are characterized by a low acceleration and high amplitude, whereas ultrasonic frequencies have an extremely high acceleration and very low amplitude. The intermediate frequencies are not considered to contribute to the mechanism of action. The acceleration associated with the low frequencies ranges between 50 and 500 m/s^2, while that associated with ultrasonic frequencies is 1400 m/s^2. The amplitudes of motion show similar differences: 5.07×10^{-3} mm at 500 Hz versus 0.555×10^{-6} mm at 800 kHz. The amplitude at 7000 Hz is 0.232×10^{-3} mm, demonstrating how quickly amplitude diminishes with increasing frequency.

To obtain a certain variability in the low-frequency range, various frequencies were selected in an approximately geometric series. Geometric series are commonly used when such experiments are done in industrial settings. Acceleration was significantly changed in only one experiment, so we can draw no far-reaching conclusions concerning the role of acceleration. Intensity (dosage) was less than 1 W/cm^2.

The following vibrations were used in the low-frequency experiments:

Frequency	Acceleration
a) 100 Hz	60 m/s^2
b) 500 Hz	50 m/s^2
c) 2500 Hz	75 m/s^2
d) 7000 Hz	500 m/s^2
e) 15000 Hz	50 m/s^2

Re a): Callus formation is clinically and radiographically improved relative to the control group. Histologic examination confirms the higher quality of the callus tissue.

Re b) and c): In the frequency range of 500–2500 Hz, where acceleration is low, a positive effect on callus formation is noted. The quality of the callus with abundant osteoblasts, calcium deposits, and cartilaginous and fibrous elements corresponds to a late stage of bone repair.

Re d): Treatment at 7 kHz demonstrates the greatest benefit yet in terms of stimulating callus tissue growth and remodeling. Compared with the other frequencies and the controls, this group shows the most advanced degree of fracture healing, which in some cases is complete.

Re e): Good callus formation is seen in comparison with the controls, although this group is surpassed by group d in terms of 3the quality and stage of healing.

For our experiments with high-frequency vibrations, we used an 800-kHz ultrasound unit and a small transducer with a radiating area of 1.4 cm^2. Years later we repeated these experiments using a low-frequency (40-kHz) ultrasound unit and found no differences in the results. The reasons for this are explained in Sect. 5.4.

Callus formation in the ultrasound-treated animals is most advanced in terms of tissue maturity compared with the other groups. The fractures show all the clinical and radiographic signs of complete union. The decidedly positive effect of ultrasound is clearly apparent and shows no dose-dependence in the energy range of 0.1 to 1.0 W/cm^2.

Fig. 34 a,b. Rabbit tibia 3 weeks after osteotomy and stable internal fixation. **a** Without ultrasound treatment, there is no X-ray evidence of callus formation. **b** In animals treated with ultrasound, the fracture is radiographically healed. The timing, duration, and intensity of the treatments were optimized in preliminary experiments

Fig. 35. a Low-power view of the specimen in Fig. 34 a. The fracture gap is partially bridged by fibroplastic and cartilaginous elements. There is no endosteal tissue reaction, and a wide interfragmental gap is present. **b** Low-power view of the specimen in Fig. 34 b. There is parosteal and endosteal callus formation, and the fracture site is consolidated

34

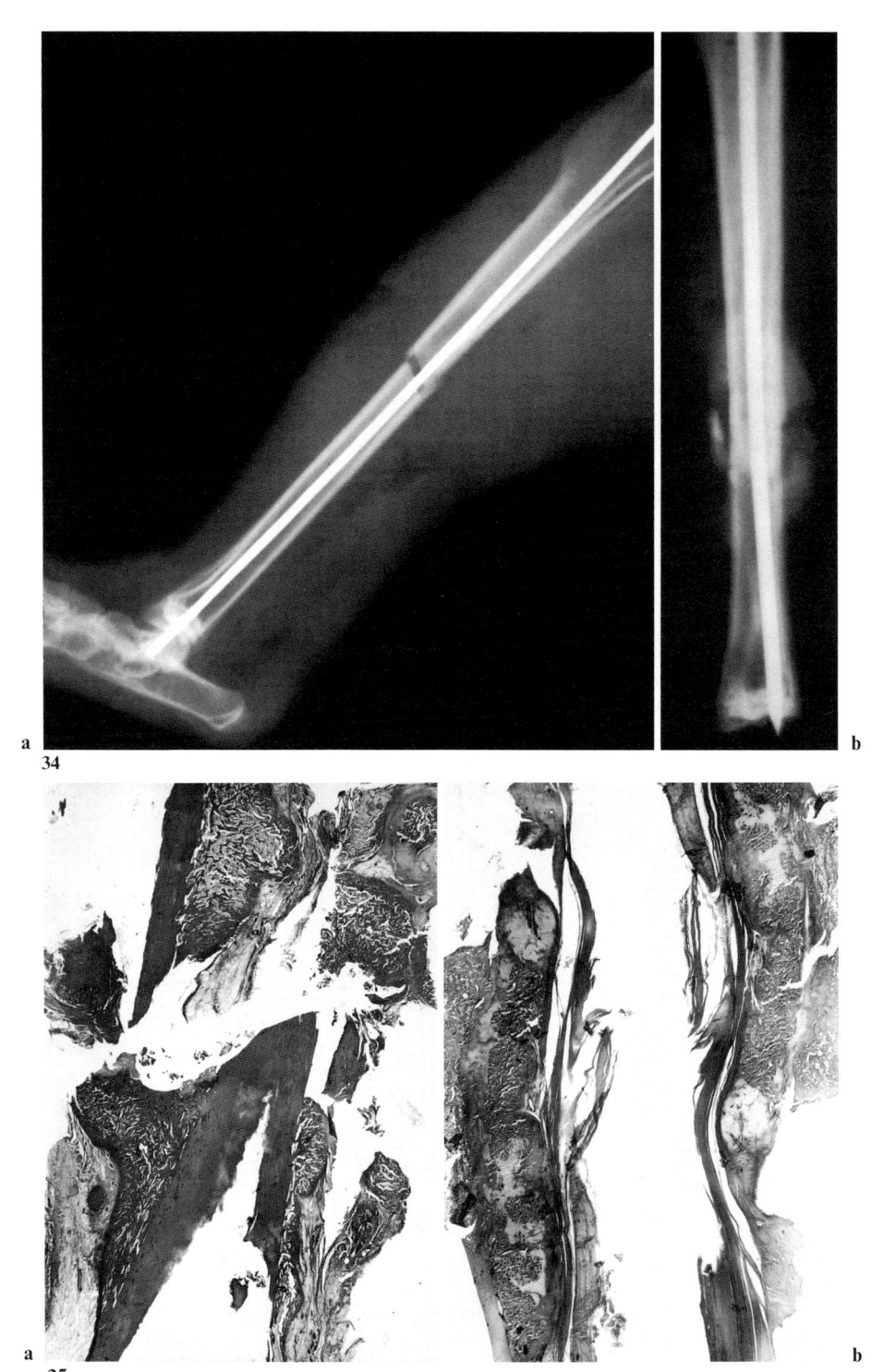

35 a b

Once a fracture has been satisfactorily immobilized, organization of the fracture hematoma occurs within 3–5 days. The invading mesenchyma, with its pluripotent capacity for differentiation, can be stimulated to more rapid growth by exposure to various mechanical stimuli. Mechanical stimulation in the form of low-level vibrations is particularly effective in inciting proliferative activity in the young, still-undifferentiated callus tissue.

When low-frequency stimulation is used, a relationship is noted between the development of callus tissue and the applied frequency. A positive response is seen in all frequency ranges, regardless of whether the fragments are rigidly immobilized or just held loosely together. Callus formation is appreciably better even at 100 Hz, and its quality increases further as higher frequencies are applied. Indeed, we found that radiographic and histologic callus improvement was frequency-dependent over the range investigated: The higher the frequency, the better the callus formation. Our experiments further demonstrate the important role of acceleration in the stimulation of tissue growth. Whereas the radiographic and histologic quality of the callus show a gradual but steady improvement as the frequency increases and acceleration remains constant, a higher rate of acceleration (e.g., 500 m/s^2 at 7 kHz or 1400 m/s^2 at 800 kHz) leads to a markedly more rapid and more differentiated callus for-

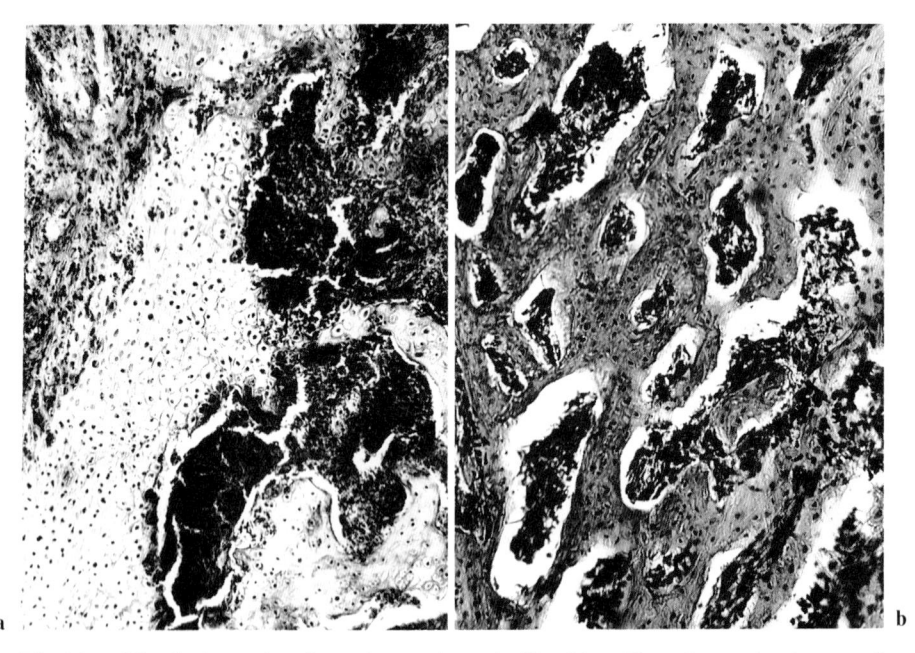

Fig. 36. a Histologic section from the specimen in Fig. 34 a. Note the predominance of granulation tissue with fibroblastic elements and cartilage cell inclusions. The histologic features correspond to the early stage of callus differentiation. **b** Histologic section from the specimen in Fig. 34 b. Besides scattered fibrous and chondromatous tissue elements, there is a predominance of osteoblasts and capillary-bound osteoid trabeculae. The heavy calcification is characteristic of healthy bone following the completion of callus formation

mation, so that the quality of callus formation at 7 kHz is comparable to that seen at ultrasonic frequencies.

From these findings we may conclude that the magnitude of the acceleration, with its potential to act upon each individual cell, is the critical factor in terms of stimulating callus formation (Figs. 34–36).

High frequency in the form of ultrasound is decidedly superior to low-frequency vibrations in its mode of action. In all cases the radiologic, clinical, and histologic assessment of callus formation demonstrates fracture healing, regardless of the postoperative stability of the fragments. Thus, the mode of action and characteristics of ultrasound energy are of crucial importance. But what is ultrasound?

5 What Is Ultrasound?

Ultrasound is the term applied to sound frequencies beyond the range of human hearing, i.e., frequencies of 20 kHz or higher. The transducers most widely used in practice are either of the magnetostrictive or piezoelectric type. The magnetostrictive effect uses magnetic energy to generate ultrasound waves by producing a cyclic change in the length of metal rods. Piezoelectric transducers generate ultrasound by the transformation of a high-frequency electrical voltage into intense mechanical vibrations. Our ultrasound therapy instruments function by the reverse piezoelectric effect (conversion of electrical to mechanical energy).

5.1 Physical Parameters

The wavelengths of ultrasound are very short. This makes it easy to emit ultrasound waves in the form of a directional, collimated beam. Measurements of sound velocity and absorption can be performed in an extremely small space. Ultrasound can be transmitted at high intensities with a large transfer of energy. The wavelength of ultrasound at 800 kHz is from 1.6 cm to 0.3×10^{-4} cm in air, 6 cm to 1.2×10^{-4} cm in liquids, and 20 cm to 4×10^{-4} cm in solids. These short wavelengths enable ultrasound to exert tissue effects at the cellular and molecular level.

Unlike light and electromagnetic waves, sound waves (and ultrasound waves) propagate in the form of longitudinal vibrations. As the wave propagates, each particle in the sound-conducting medium vibrates about the center of its resting position. The result is a transfer of energy through the medium by the alternating pressure states.

The velocity of sound propagation is a material constant and averages 1500 m/s in human tissue. The period (duration) of the vibration is frequency-dependent and is approximately one µs (700 kHz) in our therapy instruments. An ultrasound frequency of 800 kHz has proven most favorable and is presently used in most therapy units. Wavelength multiplied by frequency gives the propagation velocity. The wavelength at 800 kHz is 1.87 mm. The energy transfer depends on the transmitted sound energy measured in W/s and cm^2 and is called the acoustic intensity. A fundamental quantity in ultrasound therapy, the acoustic intensity is the critical factor determining the mechanism of action of ultrasound in tissue.

The amplitude of particle motion within an ultrasound wave is very small, is intensity-dependent, and is only 0.3 µm at 2 W/cm^2 and 800 kHz. Thus, displacements of matter within a cell do not exceed 1% of the cell diameter. The velocity of the vibrating particles of matter is frequency-independent and equals 16.5 cm/s at 2 W/cm^2. Given the high frequency of ultrasound, the vibrating particles are forced to change their direction of vibration according to the sound frequency. An extremely high acceleration of the particles is needed to accomplish this. Particle acceleration, then, is a major active force in tissues and makes significant contributions to the effects of therapeutic ultrasound.

The pressure difference between the moving particles of matter (pressure gradient) can be directly measured, depends on the particle acceleration and tissue density, and equals 8.4 atm/mm in human tissue (at 2 W/cm^2 and 800 kHz). This translates to a pressure of 0.17 atm for each cell. With each vibration this pressure alternates between a positive value (condensation) and a negative value (rarefaction) – hence the term "internal tissue massage."

The alternating acoustic pressure is a frequency-independent quantity which represents the sum of the pressure gradients and is manifested when a sound wave traveling in a homogeneous medium encounters a different tissue layer (e.g., a muscle-bone interface). The resulting reflections of the sound wave set up the alternating acoustic pressure.

As energy is transported in an ultrasound wave, some of the energy is converted to heat as a result of absorption. The absorption coefficient (decrease in sound intensity per mm tissue depth) is higher at high frequencies and depends on the conducting medium. For example, Pohlmann reports that the absorption coefficient at 800 kHz is 0.33 in muscle and 0.21 in fat. When sound propagates through a nonhomogeneous medium, the different absorption characteristics of the tissues can cause reflection of the sound wave, or the wave may be refracted. The phenomenon of the standing wave (where the incident and reflected waves are superimposed) occurs with total reflection and can increase the maximum values of the vibration by almost 100%. This leads to a dynamic distribution of the particle displacements, and all particles in the wave region are in motion. The relative displacement with respect to neighboring particles is called the deflection gradient and equals 3.3 nm for one cell at 800 kHz and 2 W/cm^2.

The results of the experimental and clinical use of therapeutic ultrasound can vary greatly depending on the applied sound intensity measured in W/cm^2, the exposure time in min, the sound frequency in kHz, the transducer radiating area in cm^2, the application technique (different sound-transmission properties of water, oils, etc., use of a stationary or moving source), the transmission mode (continuous or pulsed beam), tissue characteristics, reflections at interfaces, the formation of standing waves, and on temperature, the stage of disease, and the biologic properties of the medium. These variables can also account for the great diversity of results published during the first postwar decade.

Continuous ultrasound refers to ultrasound that is transmitted as an uninterrupted longitudinal wave, so that the applied ultrasonic energy acts continuously on the insonated medium. A continuous stress is imposed on the tissue, and there are no breaks from the "internal tissue massage." This has caused therapists to favor a moving-applicator technique over a stationary transducer. Continuous ultrasound is utilized in most therapy instruments. Although transfer of the ultrasound energy does not produce a cumulative effect (barring the formation of standing waves), problems can arise when higher doses are applied – most notably the generation of excessive heat. The use of pulsed ultrasound is an option that permits us to minimize this danger and reduce tissue stresses owing to the presence of recovery intervals between pulses.

5.2 Characteristics of Ultrasound Therapy

For decades, therapeutic ultrasound has been an integral component of physical therapy. The mechanism of action of ultrasound energy on tissues is a complex process. The effects achieved are both local and general in nature (with immediate and delayed effects) and are so varied that it is difficult to conduct a meaningful analysis of the dose-response relationship. Some mechanisms of action are known, and others can be presumed. It is quite possible that there are numerous effects with which we are not yet familiar. The mechanism of action is largely a function of intensity, frequency, exposure time, sound field, tissue type, tissue thickness, and biological variants. Intensity is the dominant factor, however.

Wiedau and Röher (1963) distinguish between the primary and secondary effects of ultrasound. The primary effects are the immediate physical and chemical changes in the sound field; they are circumscribed in their location and are measurable to some degree. Secondary effects are among the general responses of the organism based on vascular and neuroautonomic mechanisms, and thus "are a consequence of the specific characteristics of a living organism."

5.3 Types of Ultrasound

At present, three different types of therapeutic ultrasound are recognized on the basis of intensity and frequency:
a) High-frequency ultrasound: used in all areas of physiotherapy, frequency range 800–1500 kHz with intensities of 0.05–3.0 W/cm^2.
b) Low-frequency ultrasound: used in stomatology for dental calculus removal, in industry for cleaning precision parts; recently introduced into human medicine for treatment of ulcers, circulatory problems, local infections, and to stimulate fracture healing. Frequency range 40 kHz with intensities of 40–80 W/cm^2.

c) High-intensity ultrasound: used in operative medicine for dividing and uniting tissues (soft tissues and bone). Frequency range 20–40 kHz, intensity 100–200 W/cm^2.

5.4 Mechanisms of Action

We begin by considering mechanical effects, which are of primary importance due to the mechanical energy that an ultrasound beam transmits into tissues. Earlier we alluded to the pressure gradient that the longitudinal waves produce in individual cells. The tensile and compressive forces generated in the sound field exert a massage-like action which sets cellular elements into motion ("internal tissue massage"). The intensity of this internal massage can be varied as required. Therapeutic dosing at low intensity produces a weak stimulus in the tissue, which can evoke various responses in the insonated region or in the organism as a whole. Deleterious tissue effects do not occur at this level. If the dose is increased beyond 10 W/cm^2, there will be no immediate organic changes in the cells during the exposure, but this level may be sufficient for the onset of cavitation. Greater amounts of energy will cause damage to cell populations or even to whole organs. These secondary lesions are irreversible, and they can be demonstrated histologically in soft tissues and radiographically in bone. Thus we are dealing with two opposing mechanisms of action, depending on the intensity of the exposure: (1) "internal tissue massage" at very low levels, which promotes cellular metabolism, regeneration, blood flow, and tissue oxygen delivery, and (2) the destruction of tissues or small organs at high dose levels. For practical purposes, then, intensities of 0.05–2.0 W/cm^2 are indicated for ordinary conservative ultrasound therapy, while 100–200 W/cm^2 would be appropriate for some surgical indications.

It has been clearly established that low-frequency ultrasound – generally applied by immersion in a medicated or unmedicated water bath – has the same mechanism of action in tissue as high-frequency ultrasound. Low-frequency ultrasound has a very long wavelength that carries a large amount of energy. When these long waves come in contact with the medium to be treated, they are refracted, and cavitation occurs at the interface. This mechanism is utilized for the painless removal of pathologic tissue (in ulcerations), and the massaging action improves the microcirculation (increased pO_2 can be measured transcutaneously). Bacteria and fungi are destroyed. A large portion of the ultrasound energy penetrates into the tissue (0.1–0.3 W/cm^2) and exerts the same effects produced by high-frequency ultrasound. Thus, low-frequency ultrasound is useful for the stimulation of fracture healing, and it offers the advantages of improving blood flow and oxygen delivery to the affected body part, eliminating local infections and ulcerations, and providing a route for the transcutaneous administration of medications.

Besides mechanical effects, thermal effects are a fundamental property of therapeutic ultrasound. Following the principle of "where there is motion there is heat," the thermal effects of ultrasound result from the vibrational motion imparted to particles of matter in the cell, leading to the conversion of kinetic energy into heat. The energy intensity of the beam decreases rapidly with increasing tissue depth as a result of absorption. The interaction between mechanical and thermal effects can be described by the absorption coefficient. This coefficient is tissue-specific and shows us how much mechanical energy is converted (lost) to heat generation as the beam travels through various tissues. The heating effect is intensity-dependent and is negligible at low dose levels but can become significant at levels of just $2-5$ W/cm^2. Our studies indicate that significant tissue heating does not occur at a dose of 0.1 W/cm^2.

Kihn (1956) found that ultrasound exposure at therapeutic levels (1 W/cm^2) did not raise the temperature of the insonated skin. He also showed that therapeutic ultrasound increases the rate of oxygen diffusion (without heating) in the treated tissue. His hypothesis that an ultrasound stimulus in the therapeutic range increases the permeability of cell membranes, leading to increased metabolic processes within the cell itself, and can produce this effect with no associated change in cutaneous blood flow is consistent with numerous observations by other authors (Nödl 1949; Lehmann et al. 1967; Baumann and Presch 1950; etc.).

Other effects of ultrasound are based on physicochemical mechanisms. Chemical effects are often linked to "cavitation," a process involving the expansion or rupture of gas pockets by the large tensile stresses exerted by the ultrasound waves. Cavitation occurs when a large amount of energy ($\geq$ 10 W/cm^2) is transmitted into the tissue, and the cavitation associated with high-intensity ultrasound can cause irreversible damage. At therapeutic levels, tiny bubbles are formed that do not harm the insonated medium. Wiedau and Röher (1963) report that cavitation does not occur in living tissue exposed to low ultrasound doses, claiming that such events are ruled out by "the frequency and intensity dependence of cavitation, the strength of the macroscopic cell structure, and the viscosity of the tissue fluid."

Certain chemical reactions are known to occur in insonated tissues. These include changes in the diffusibility of various substances through membranes or through the intact skin. Changes from the gel and sol state can be induced by ultrasound. The conductivity of electrolytic solutions is increased, oxidative processes are initiated, and chemical reactions proceed as under catalytic conditions. Additionally, ultrasound can shift pH values toward alkalinity, release certain pharmacologic substances, and accelerate fluid uptake in tissues.

Besides the mechanical, thermal, and chemical effects of ultrasound, which incidentally are interrelated and cannot occur in isolation from one another, it is useful to consider "biological effects" based upon the response of isolated organs and the organism as a whole. This response represent the sum of the foregoing mechanisms of action and possibly of other, previously unknown factors and is a result of neurohormonal interactions, particularly with regard to effects on the neural end-plates. These biological effects of ultrasound are of major practical importance and form the basis for therapeutic applications. Any change in physical parameters such as frequency, intensity, or exposure time leads to changes in the associated mechanical, thermal, and chemical effects, resulting in an altered biological response. This biologic mechanism of action can also be interpreted as the effect of the exposure on the organism as a whole. This would be consistent with previously described therapeutic effects, our own experience, and with the principle of always viewing the organism as a integral whole.

Effects on the autonomic nervous system are of primary importance in this regard. Schliephake (1949) and Kohlrausch (1955) were able to demonstrate the effect of vibrations on the autonomic nervous system. Other effects have been demonstrated by chronaximetry, electromyographic studies, thermal measurements in terminal vessels (Otto 1955), and studies on the release of acetylcholine and histamine in tissue (Busnel et al. 1954). The mechanisms of these effects operate by cutivisceral and cerebrospinal pathways and can be demonstrated by observing functional changes in internal organs such as the stomach (Wiedau and Röher 1963).

According to Pospisilova (1973), ultrasound can influence connective tissue metabolism in vivo in complex ways: It accelerates the formation of specific cells, influences polysaccharide metabolism, acts homeostatically to balance collagen metabolism in the synthesis phase, and also affects collagen lysis (probably by the activation of collagenase).

Kihn (1956) characterized these complex mechanisms of action as a nonspecific stimulus response. Wiedau and Röher (1963) believe that the functional state of the autonomic nervous system is "retuned" in the direction of sedation, emphasizing the central inhibitory effect on specific tonus centers. Wiedau and Röfher (1963) also mention the spasmolytic effect of ultrasound, the inhibition of sympathetic pathways that mediate pain sensation, and muscular relaxation. The principal locus of action appears to be at neural endplates.

5.5 The Piezoelectric Effect in Bone

An extremely important mechanism of action of ultrasound is based on the demonstrable presence of electrical potentials in bone. These potentials, which are always present physiologically, are potentiated by exposure to ultrasonic energy. This fact has a fundamental bearing on the stimulation of bone tissue, and it explains why the stimulation of fracture healing by electric current (electrical stimulation) and by ultrasound exposure (ultrasound stimulation) are not competitive but have the same principle of action. It is of secondary importance whether fracture healng is stimulated by electrical or ultrasonic energy. However, the use of ultrasound offers some definite advantages: ultrasound equipment is available everywhere and has a variety of applications; the treatment is simple, and there are no complications.

Friedenberg and Kohanin (1968) demonstrated that live, nonstressed bone carries a permanent direct-current polarization that depends on the activity of the bone cells: Areas with high cellular activity (metaphyses) are electronegative in relation to less metabolically active sites (diaphyses). A bioelectrical potential of 1–15 mV, resulting from perfusion of the bone by the electrically charged blood, has been measured from the bone surface in rabbits (Weigert 1978, Schellnak et al. 1979).

The piezoelectric properties of bone, discovered by Fukada and Yasuda in 1957, refer to the appearance of electrical potentials in bone acted upon by mechanical tension, compression, shear stress, or torsion. When a bone is mechanically deformed, two opposite charges develop at the ends of its electrical axis. Areas under compression become electronegative, while areas under tension become electropositive. Basset (1965), Cieszynski (1973), Lechner (1976), and Becker and Bachmann (1965) believe that piezoelectricity results from the mechanical shearing action of fibrils and collagen fibers with an associated deformation of molecular hydrogen bonds. The measurable potential is 0.5–3 mV and is proportional to the magnitude of the applied stress (Kraus 1978).

Besides the maximum negative potential at the fracture site, the entire affected bone exhibits a relative increase in electronegativity (Karus 1974; Weigert 1978). The fracture potentials, injury potentials, or stress-induced potentials are most likely attributable to metabolic and physicochemical processes. The fracture hematoma, with its local change in pH, also must play a role.

We were able to demonstrate the following: The planum cutaneum in the middle third of the tibia was surgically exposed in supine rabbits under hexobarbital anesthesia. Two nonpolarized silver chloride electrodes were secured to the flat tibial surface, stripped of periosteum, with Perlon threads and wetted with 0.9% NaCl. The contact area between the electrodes and tibial cortex was 0.75 cm^2, and the electrodes were spaced 50 mm apart. Both electrodes were connected by shielded leads to a digital voltmeter (G-1001.500, VEB Funkwerk Erfurt) which measured the basic potential of the bone, its ohmic resistance, and the potential and resistance changes during ultrasound exposure. The experimental animal and the digital voltmeter were grounded. Following

Table 2. Piezoelectric effect in the intact and fractured rabbit tibia, with and without ultrasound (see Sect. 6.3)

Basic potential in intact bone [in mV]	$\bar{x}$	SD
Without ultrasound (US)	−11.4	0.6
With US at 0.2 W/cm^2	−11.7	0.7
Fracture without US, day 21	−12.5	0.4
Fracture with US at 0.2 W/cm^2	−13.4	0.4

Ohmic resistance in intact bone [in $\Omega \cdot$ mm]	$\bar{x}$	SD
Without US	5.8	0.45
With US at 0.2 W/cm^2	5.5	0.51
Fracture without US, day 21	5.43	0.4
Fracture with US at 0.2 W/cm^2	5.19	0.4

measurement of the basic potential and ohmic resistance, the bone was insonated over the coat of the proximal tibia. Measurements were performed in 11 rabbits; the results are shown in Table 2.

An increase in the direct-current potential on the fractured tibia was detected 8 s after insonation commenced. The potential increase became maximal at 21 s and remained at that level throughout the exposure. Nine seconds after the ultrasound was turned off, the potential returned to the initial value. Exposure was maintained for 3 min. Even with a longer insonation time, the same potential increase by an average of 0.9 mV was recorded. When the intensity was increased to 1 W/cm^2, the 0.9-mV potential increase remained constant while the ohmic resistance fell by 0.2 Ω. The potential increase during ultrasound exposure was consistently reproducible.

Impedance Measurement

Measurement of the electrical impedance of the callus tissue is of interest in this context. The condition of membranes in tissue structures can be investigated by passive electrical methods. Here it is assumed that a biologic membrane has the electrical properties of a dissipative capacitor. The membrane consists of two protein layers separated by a lipid layer which has a high resistance compared with the surrounding electrolytes and functions as a dielectric. The porosity and intrinsic conductivity of the lipids allow for direct-current conductivity through the membrane. According to these concepts, the passive electrical characteristics of the membrane can be represented by an equivalent circuit consisting of a resistance R_p with a capacitor C and a series resistor R_r.

The electrical impedance of a cellular suspension or an arrangement of membranes like that occurring in tissue represents the sum of the impedances of the individual membranes. It is important to note that in this case the electric current developing in response to an applied voltage no longer flows just perpendicular to the membrane surface but also tangentially. The charged membrane surface and the medium interact to form an electrical "double layer" whose charges can be displaced in the alternating electric field, permitting tangential conduction to occur.

The equivalent circuit diagram of a tissue fragment placed between two electrodes is highly complex. However, because the different tissue membranes have similar equivalent circuit diagrams, the system can be described by the parallel arrangement of two series circuits with capacitors and two resistors. From measurements of electrical impedance, inferences can be drawn regarding the functional state and maturity of the callus and the load-bearing capacity of the fracture. This is why we considered it important to measure electrical impedance during tibial fracture healing.

Of the three methods available for measuring electrical impedance, the analysis of rectangular pulse distortion is best suited for the investigation of callus and bone. The analysis is performed using a bioimpedance measuring instrument.

We inserted a pair of sharp measuring electrodes made of V_2A steel into the periosteal callus to a depth of 3 mm, spacing them 10 mm apart. The sensitive surface area was 4 mm^2. A constant temperature of 23 °C was maintained in the examination room. The amplitude of the rectangular input pulse was set to a constant scale value of 25 mm. The frequency was 80 kHz. Distortion of the rectangular pulse caused by its passage through the callus was displayed on an oscillograph (type EO 174 N) and read on the millimeter scale. We measured the amplitude height H and the amount of pulse distortion h. The distortion is illustrated in Fig. 37.

Measurements of H in 40 bones (rabbit dry tibial cortex) indicated a mean value of 3 mm (SD 1 mm). The amount of pulse distortion h averaged 1 mm (SD 1 mm). The results of the measurements are shown in Tables 3 and 4.

In experimental group II, measurements on days 21, 28, and 42 postfracture indicated a significantly smaller decrease in the amplitude height H than in group I. The parameter h changed significantly in group II on days 21 and 28.

In impedance measurements the rectangular pulse is distorted by the specific passive electrical behavior of the callus tissue. The H values are changed in accordance with the age of the fracture. The higher the water content of the callus tissue and the lower its mineral content, the smaller the degree of pulse distortion. Increasing mineralization reduces the electrical conductivity of the callus while increasing its capacitive and ohmic resistance. The greatest pulse distortion is produced by normal bone.

In summary, it may be said that the direct-current potential resident in the bone is increased by 0.9 ($\pm$ 0.4) mV during ultrasound irradiation of the fractured tibia. The potential increase becomes maximal 21 s after the treatment is started, and this value persists throughout the exposure. The potential returns to its initial value 9 s after the exposure is terminated. The potential

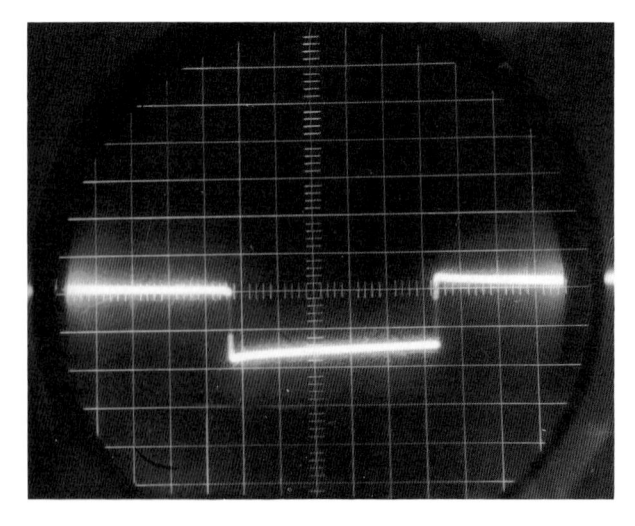

Fig. 37. Distortion of a rectangular pulse by the passive electrical behavior of the callus tissue

Ultrasound Conductivity

Table 3. Amplitude height H of callus tissue during fracture healing (see Sect. 6.3)

Days postfracture	Group I [mm]			Group II [mm]			t value
	n	x̄	SD	n	x̄	SD	
7	10	13	1				
14	10	18	6				
21	10	16	3	10	22	2	5.81
28	10	12	3	15	18	2	9.33
42	16	12	3	12	10	1	3.09
70	16	10	3	14	12	1	1.97
126	17	7	3	17	9	5	2.19
168	10	4	1	10	4	1	1.93

Table 4. Degree of pulse distortion during fracture healing (see Sect. 6.2)

Days postfracture	Group I [mm]			Group II [mm]			t value
	n	x̄	SD	n	x̄	SD	
7	10	2	1				
14	10	4	1				
21	10	2	2	10	2	2	15.81
28	15	2	2	15	3	2	8.21
42	15	2	1	15	2	1	0.00
70	12	2	1	15	2	1	1.44
126	16	1	1	16	1	1	0.29
168	10	1	1	10	1	1	0.00

increase is reproducible. The ohmic resistance of the fractured bone does not decrease significantly during ultrasound exposure.

Ultrasound waves are longitudinal pressure waves that deform the collagen fibrils, collagen fibers, apatite crystals, and all callus cells present in the sound field. Conversion of the mechanical energy into a piezoelectric potential is another primary effect of the ultrasound waves. The resulting piezoelectricity acts through electrochemical mechanisms to exert a stimulatory effect on the osteoprogenitor cells.

5.6 Ultrasound Conductivity

Ultrasound conductivity is of fundamental importance in the therapeutic application of ultrasound. Water immersion treatment with ultrasound is a well known procedure in physical therapy. Different media in the body differ greatly in their absorption of ultrasonic energy. The following experiment was performed to demonstrate the ultrasound conductivity of bone tissue: In 20 rabbits the distal third of the tibia was fractured and stabilized by internal fixation (Kirschner wire). In 10 of the animals, insonation of the proximal tibia was commenced starting on the 6th day postfracture. After 3 weeks all 10 of the ultrasound-treated fractures were solid, while the 10 bones not treated with ultrasound still exhibited gross motion at the fracture site and showed no radiographic signs of consolidation.

Measurements in Experimental Animals

The absorption of ultrasound energy was measured as follows: The proximal end of the tibia was insonated in 10 rabbits (beam area 1.4 cm^2, intensity 0.05–0.1 W/cm^2). A second transducer with a receiving area of 1.4 cm^2 was used to record the transmitted energy. It was placed over the posterior tibial surface, on the foot, and over the femur and was connected to the EO 174 A oscillograph. Ultrasound waves striking the barium titanate crystals in the receiving transducer mechanically deform the crystals in the rhythm of the ultrasound waves. The piezoelectric response of the crystals generates extremely small potential differences that can be displayed on the oscillograph and measured in mV.

Findings: Sound intensity arriving at the flexor surface of the tibia relative to the applied intensity of 0.05–0.1 W/cm^2: proximal tibia 2%–3.5%, hip joint 0.5%–2%, distal tibia 1%–6%, dorsum of foot 0.5%–1.5%, ankle joint 1%–2%.

The same intensities were measured when the positions of the transmitting and receiving transducers were interchanged. The ultrasound propagates in all directions and through all tissue layers, including the bones and joints. The sound field encompasses the entire posterior extremity.

When the femur is insonated at 0.05 W/cm^2 through the coat of the extensor surface, 0.2% of the source intensity can still be measured on the denuded cortex of the tibial diaphysis with a transmitter-receiver separation of 12 cm. When intensities of 0.05, 0.2, 0.4, and 1.0 W/cm^2 are applied to a pedicled muscle flap measuring 20 × 20 × 10 mm in size, the corresponding ultrasound absorption is 60%, 55%, 50%, and 40%.

The degrees of absorption measured in a 20 × 20 × 20-mm vascularized flap of skin, muscle, and bone insonated at 0.05, 0.2, 0.4, and 1.0 W/cm^2 are 96%, 95%, 93%, and 90% (Table 5).

Table 5. Intensity loss through a live skin-muscle-bone flap (tibia) 2 × 2 × 2 cm in size. The upper surface was insonated, and intensity was measured on the lower surface

Intensity [W/cm^2]	Ultrasound absorption [%]	Received sound intensity [%]
0.05	96	4
0.2	95	5
0.4	93	7
1.0	90	10

Measurements in Humans

In 20 healthy human subjects of both sexes ranging from 25 to 55 years of age, ultrasound was applied at various sites on the upper arm and forearm, and intensities were measured at various distances from those sites. The radiating area of the transmitting transducer was 1.4 cm^2, the intensity 0.05–0.7 W/cm^2. The receiving transducer has a sensitive area of 1.4 cm^2 and was connected to an EO 174 A oscillograph, which gives a visual display of minute potential differences and a quantitative readout in mV. These values were converted to intensity in W/cm^2. The basic principle of the process is as follows: Ultrasound waves from the transmitter strike the barium titanate crystals of the receiving transducer and mechanically deform them, generating piezoelectric voltage signals that have the same rhythm as the incident ultrasound waves.

We found that when the proximal third of the upper arm was insonated at 0.7 W/cm^2, an intensity of 0.023 W/cm^2 could be measured at a distance of 18.7 cm (humeral condyle). An intensity of 0.0059 W/cm^2 was measured at a distance of 30 cm (middle third of forearm) (see Fig. 37).

These experiments confirm the propagation of ultrasound energy through organs while underscoring the high acoustic conductivity of bone. This has important practical implications: The fracture does not always have to be insonated directly, and the cast does not always have to be windowed over the fracture site. It is feasible to apply ultrasound away from the fracture site, though this requires the use of a higher intensity.

6 Animal Experiments

6.1 The Rabbit as an Animal Model

As Urist and Johnson (1943) point out, fracture healing in man does not differ essentially from that in other mammals. This accounts for the very frequent use of small mammals, especially rabbits, in experimental studies on callus formation and fracture healing.

Because the growth rate of rabbits is approximately 40 times greater than in humans, a 200-day-old rabbit corresponds roughly in age to a 22-year-old human. Rabbits are fully mature at 11–12 months; their epiphyseal growth plates are closed (Jäger and Gördes 1976). Animals of this age have an average weight of 3 kg. Rabbit bones are more brittle than human bones, and bone healing progresses at a faster rate. The long bones of the extremities have approximately the same structure, however (Demeter and Matyas 1928; Kurz 1981). The weight of all air-dried bones in the rabbit equals 7%–8.3% of the live weight. The weight of the extremities accounts for 50% of the total air-dried bone weight. One-third of the bone weight consists of organic substances, two-thirds of inorganic substances (Schwarze 1979).

In our experiments we used mongrel rabbits obtained from one breeder. The animals were fed identical diets and kept in identical cages. The age at the start of the experiments was 190 days, the average weight 3 kg ($\pm$ 0.4 kg).

6.2 Experimental Method

Following the induction of intravenous anesthesia through an ear vein, a tibial fracture was produced in all animals. In 100 rabbits this was done by operatively exposing the bone and osteotomizing it with a fine chisel or saw, and in 200 by fracturing the closed limb over a fulcrum. All open fractures were stabilized at once by internal fixation. Kirschner wires of varying diameters were used, so that some of the fractures were rigidly immobilized while others were moderately stabilized (casting was not performed). The closed fractures were reduced and immobilized in a long leg cast with the knee and ankle joints in functional positions.

Twenty-six of the 300 animals were lost due to various causes (osteomyclitis 9, anesthetic death 6, fat embolism 3, dog bite 2, unknown cause 6), so that 274 animals were available for evaluation. Since 48 of the animals had bilateral closed tibial fractures, 322 fractures were available for study. Two experimental groups were formed:

Group I: A control group with 135 fractures not treated with ultrasound. All values of the investigated parameters for specific points in time are drawn from this group.

Group II: 187 fractures treated with ultrasound.

6.3 Statistical Evaluation

For statistical evaluation of the data derived from a subpopulation under equal conditions, the sample size (n), arithmetic mean (x), and standard deviation (a) are calculated.

For the simple comparison of mean values, it is assumed that ranges are available for a random quantity Y from normally distributed, independent samples with unknown expected values and variances.

The random samples $x_i \ldots x_n$ and $y_i \ldots y_n$ are each drawn from two subpopulations that are to be compared. The object is to test the null hypothesis H_0 that both expected values are equal: $EX = EY$.

In the case of equal variances ($D^2 X = D^2 Y$), the t value is calculated by:

$$t = \frac{\bar{x} - \bar{y}}{\sqrt{(n-1)s_x^2 + (m-1)s_y^2}} \cdot \sqrt{\frac{(n+m-2)nm}{n+m}}$$

where x is the mean value of the variables X, i.e. whose range is $(x_i \ldots x_n)$, y is the mean value of the variables Y, i.e. whose range is $(y_i \ldots y_n)$, and s_x^2 and s_y^2 are the empirical variances of the variables x and y. The double t test is used to determine whether the hypothesis must be rejected or retained. The test is two-tailed with a 0.05 level of significance ($\alpha = 5\%$).

The condition for rejection is

$$|t| > t_{n+m-2,\, 1-\alpha/2}.$$

The values are compared with the tabulated values of the t distribution. A probability of error less than 5% ($p < 0.05$) is regarded as statistically significant. The statistical evaluation of trait values and the frequency of their occurrence is accomplished by a two-dimensional frequency analysis.

7 Effect of Ultrasound on Fracture Callus

Callus comprises the intermediate stage in the healing of a fracture toward soundness. The detection of healthy callus tissue in a fracture treated with ultrasound forms the basis for proving the stimulatory efect of ultrasound. To furnish this proof, the following investigations were performed:
- Radiographic studies
- Strength tests
- Histologic studies, scanning electron microscopy
- Bone scintigraphy
- Angiographic studies
- Biochemical studies
- Total mineral analysis
- Sequential polychrome labeling
- Temperature measurements
- Summary of findings

7.1 Radiographic Studies

In the control group of animals whose tibial fracture was either fixed with an intramedullary Kirschner wire or immobilized in plaster, faint callus shadow is visible on radiographs at 3 weeks. A wide interfragmental gap is still present at this stage. Callus formation appears predominantly as periosteal callus; the fracture is not healed.

The following radiographic features are characteristic of secondary fracture healing:
- an appositional callus cuff or periosteal collar bridging the fracture site,
- almost no endosteal callus formation,
- initially little or no involvement of the cortical ends in callus formation,
- irritative callus and resorption zones in the region of interfragmental contact,
- development of a fixation callus.

Radiographs of the tibia and fibula were taken in the anterior, posterior, and mediolateral projections after the animals were killed, the limb amputated, and the soft tissues removed. The films were evaluated for callus development, interfragmental gap, and mineralization. The findings are summarized in Tables 6–8.

Radiographic Studies

Table 6. Radiographic assessment of callus development. (*1* No callus, *2* faint callus development at the immediate level of the fracture, *3* spindle-shaped or rounded callus confined largely to the fracture site, *4* massive spindle-shaped callus extending well past the fracture site proximally and distally)

Days postfracture	Group I Prevalence of findings [%]					Group II Prevalence of findings [%]				
	n	1	2	3	4	n	1	2	3	4
7	16	44	56							
14	16		94	6						
21	16		56	44		16		26	75	
28	16		25	75		16		6	94	
42	16			69	31	16			50	50
70	16			56	44	16			38	62
126	16				100	16				100

Table 7. Radiographic assessment of the fracture gap. (*1* Gap clearly visible, *2* gap partially bridged, *3* gap completely bridged)

Days postfracture	Group I Prevalence of findings [%]			Group II Prevalence of findings		
	1	2	3	1	2	3
7	100					
14	100					
21	75	25		75	25	
28	56	44		38	62	
42	12	50	38	0	50	50
70		25	75		12	88
126			100			100
168			100			100

Table 8. Radiographic assessment of mineralization. (*1* No mineralization, *2* incipient mineralization, *3* advanced mineralization, *4* complete mineralization)

Days postfracture	Group I Prevalence of findings [%]					Group II Prevalence of findings [%]				
	n	1	2	3	4	n	1	2	3	4
7	16	75	4							
14	16	38	62							
21	16		81	19		16		69	31	
28	16		63	37		16		38	62	
42	16		19	56	25	16		6	50	44
70	16			38	62	16			12	88
126	16			6	94	16				100
168	16				100					100

load in the three-point bending test was determined under standardized conditions. The test data were synchronously recorded with an XY plotter, which showed deflection as a function of applied load.

Calculations: The formula for a solid rod in solid-state mechanics served as the basis for calculating the bending strength σ_z of the callus under a three-point bending load:

$$\delta_z \text{ callus} = \frac{1 \cdot F}{\pi \cdot R^3} \frac{N}{mm^2}$$

The bending strength δ_z of the cortex and compact bone was calculated using the formula for a hollow cylinder:

$$\delta_B \text{ compact} = \frac{1 \cdot F}{4\pi \cdot R_A^2 (R_A - R_I)} \frac{N}{mm^2}$$

In these formulas l is the distance between the points of support (62 mm), R is the radius of the callus cross section in mm, F is the maximum fracture load in newtons, R_A is the outer radius of the tibial cross section at the center of the diaphysis in mm, and R_I is the inner radius of the tibial cross section (without the cortex and compact bone) at the center of the tibia in mm.

In determining the bending strength δ_B of the compact bone, the bone was regarded as a standard cylinder whose radius is a mean value. Fifty tibial cross sections in the middle third of the diaphysis were measured in the anteroposterior dimension. The mean value of the tibial cross sections was 8.05 mm, with a mean cortical/compact bone thickness of 1.4 mm.

The maximum fracture load of a healthy unfractured tibia (cortex) averages 351.63 N based on studies in a total of 24 tibias. The results are summarized in Table 9.

The bending strength of the unfractured tibia (compact bone) averages 91.7 based on studies in 23 bones. These results are shown in Table 10.

The maximum fracture load on days 42 and 70 postfracture is significantly greater in group II than in group I, where the fracture load does not approach

Table 9. Maximum fracture load of the fractured tibia as a function of time

Days postfracture	Group I [N]			Group II [N]			t value
	n	x̄	SD	n	x̄	SD	
14	11	140.63	23.13				
21	10	190.57	27.12	11	195.00	25.11	0.19
28	11	283.33	48.81	11	298.81	20.10	0.36
42	12	309.25	30.97	12	375.82	29.12	3.22
70	9	311.42	40.50	15	399.42	44.28	3.85
126	9	324.11	65.38	9	366.24	68.42	1.48
168	7	361.61	34.48	8	360.12	57.27	0.06

Table 10. Bending strength δB of the compact bone during fracture healing

Days postfracture	Group I [N]			Group II [N]			t value
	n	x̄	SD	n	x̄	SD	
14	11	27.14	10.98				
21	10	41.67	9.92	10	45.55	8.9	0.23
28	8	68.19	9.79	11	77.19	14.42	1.53
42	12	69.85	1.15	11	81.42	11.84	3.37
70	9	75.31	18.11	12	90.55	13.56	2.31
126	9	70.51	20.49	15	71.87	10.69	0.23
168	7	86.25	10.21	7	89.67	15.18	0.33

the 70-day value in group II until day 126. The fracture load in group II corresponds to the fracture load of the unfractured tibia.

The bending strength of the callus on day 70 is significant greater than the values calculated for group I. On day 126 the bending strength of the callus is approximately equal in both groups. When calculations are based on the formula for a hollow cylinder, the bending strength in group II on days 40 and 70 is significantly higher than in group I.

The bending strength σ_B of the compact bone in group II reaches its highest value on day 70 postfracture, which corresponds to that of an unfractured tibia. The bending strength on day 70 postfracture in group II approximates the value measured on day 126 in group I.

7.3 Histologic Studies, Scanning Electron Microscopy

Histologic examination of the control group following 3 weeks' immobilization of the tibial fracture shows abundant granulation tissue with predominantly fibroplastic elements. At this stage there are no more signs of residual hematoma except for a few scattered deposits of iron pigment. The fracture gap contains abundant cartilaginous tissue, with only half of cases showing capillary-bound osteoid trabeculae. Calcium deposits are extremely rare, as are osteoblastic elements. The callus tissue is confined largely to the periosteum. There is maximum mobilization of mesenchymal tissue.

The histomorphology of fracture healing during conservative treatment follows the pattern of secondary bone healing:
- formation of a fracture hematoma;
- coagulation and organization of the hematoma through the ingrowth of granulation and fibrovascular tissue;
- activation of osteoprogenitor cells and their stages of differentiation in the osteogenic series (preosteoblast, young osteoblast, mature osteoblast, young osteocyte, mature osteocyte) by osteoinductive substances;
- conversion to fibrous connective-tissue callus;

- formation of fiber bone by enchondral (compressive and shear forces) and membranous (tensile forces) ossification;
- formation of lamellar bone, reinforcement of the fiber-bone scaffold by lamellar bone deposition;
- functional remodeling of the compact bone by regeneration of the osteons.

In each of 151 rabbit tibial fractures, we performed four histologic examinations of the decalcified callus-bone specimen. Two of the sections from each fracture were stained with hematoxylin-eosin, and two with azocarmine-aniline blue orange (azan).

As Table 11 shows, a two-dimensional frequency analysis of the histomorphologic criteria in each experimental group indicated a significantly higher prevalence of criteria 3 and 4 in group II on days 42, 70, and 126 postfracture compared with group I. The histomorphologic differentiation following ultrasound fracture treatment shows a more advanced degree of callus maturity. The greater abundance of osteoblasts and the stronger activation of osteoblastic activity are especially noteworthy.

Scanning electron microscopic examinations were performed in 18 fractures as follows:

Transverse bone-callus sections 3 mm thick were sawed from the fracture site and fixed to a metal block with Duosan adhesive. In some specimens the inorganic constituents were dissolved with 5% nitric acid. The specimens were vapor coated with a thin conductive carbon layer and examined with the JEOL JSM-S1 scanning electron microscope (Electronic Optics Laboratory, Tokyo) using an accelerating voltage of 4 kV. The number of examinations are shown in Table 12. Evaluation of the photomicrographs (Figs. 39–41) confirm the favorable effect of ultrasound exposure.

7.4 Bone Scintigraphy

Bone scintigraphy is based on the detection of the uptake of bone-seeking radiopharmaceuticals at specific sites in bone. The rate and intensity of radiotracer uptake depend on the local metabolic state and perfusion of the bone.

We perform bone scintigraphy with technetium-99m hydroxyethylidene diphosphonate (HEDP). This study is useful for investigating the physiologic changes that accompany fracture healing (Becker et al. 1974; Bessler 1970; Kleditzsch 1980). Bone lesions present as areas of increased tracer uptake.

Fig. 39. a Group I, 3 weeks p.f.: disordered, clumpy ground substance with scattered collagen fibers (90 ×). **b** Group II, 3 weeks p.f.: abundant collagen fiber network showing fiber alignment (90 ×)

Fig. 40. a Group I, 4 weeks p.f.: diffuse, clumpy bone substance showing incipient mineralization (90 ×). **b** Group II, 4 weeks p.f.: directional collagen fibers with pronounced mineralization (90 ×)

39 a, b

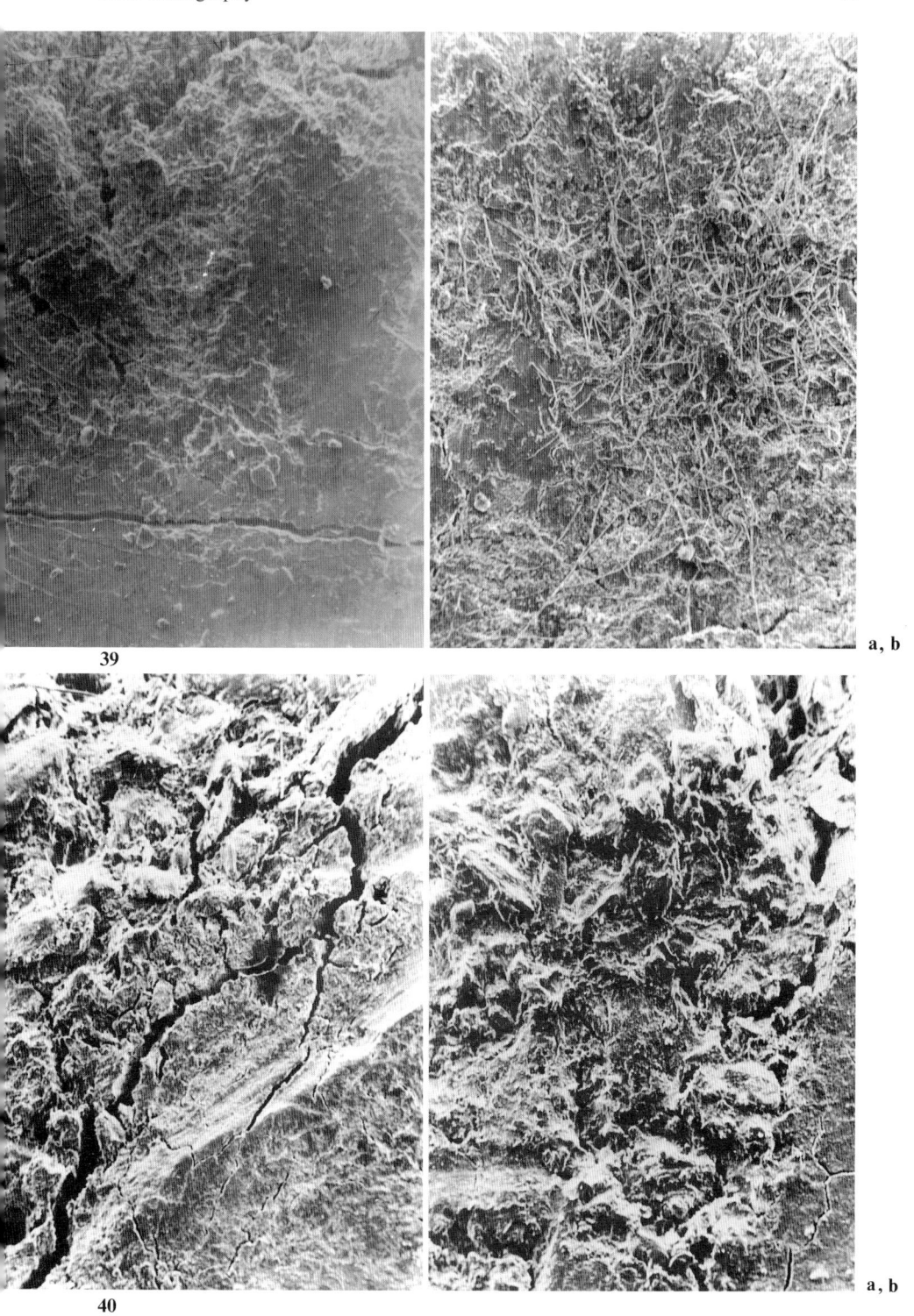

40 a, b

Table 11. Micromorphologic criteria for evaluating tissue differentiation with and without therapeutic ultrasound.
(*1* Undifferentiated callus tissue with immature multinucleated cartilage cells; *2* finely trabecular, spikelike periosteal fiber bone with considerable cartilaginous and fibrous callus and normal osteoblastic activity; *3* massive fiber bone with broad trabeculae, few mature cartilage cells, markedly increased osteoblastic activity with an increased number of osteoblasts; *4* lamellar bone with well-developed haversian systems)

Days postfracture	Group I Prevalence of criteria [%]					Group II Prevalence of criteria [%]				
	n	1	2	3	4	n	1	2	3	4
7	7	70	30							
14	8	37.5	62.5							
21	10	10	80	10		10		60	40	
28	12		50	50		12		25	75	
42	18		24	76		20		6.6	66.6	26.7
70	12		16.6	83.4		12			50	50
126	10			20	80	10				100
168	5				100	5				100

Table 12. Number of electron microscopic examinations in both experimental groups

Days postfracture	Number of animals	
	Group I	Group II
21	2	2
28	2	2
42	5	5

Rarely the scans demonstrate "cold spots," which may be caused by occlusion of the intramedullary vessels.

Bone scintigraphy is a valuable method for monitoring the course of fracture healing and assessing the biological activity of a fracture (Bessler 1970; Becker et al. 1974; Unterspann and Fink 1981). The following specific questions are at issue:

– What quantitative changes in tracer uptake occur during the course of fracture healing?
– Are there differences in the mean count rates per unit area in the two experimental groups at equal points in time?
– When is fracture healing scintigraphically complete?
– Does the scintigram always indicate fracture healing when there is conclusive X-ray and clinical evidence that full consolidation has occurred?

The animals were placed under hexobarbital anesthesia for the radiotracer injection. Forty-five minutes after the i.v. injection of 8 MBq ^{99m}Tc diphosphonate/kg body weight, an average of 100.000 counts were recorded from both extremities. The scintigraphic examination was performed using a stan-

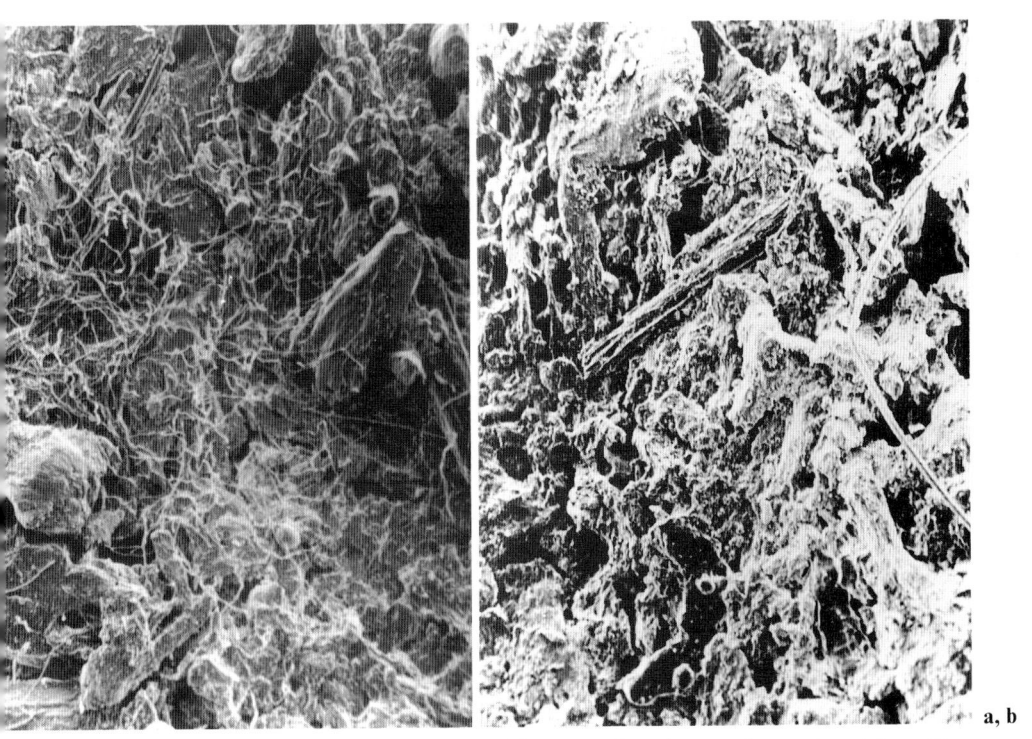

Fig. 41. a Group I, 6 weeks p.f.: collagen fibers not aligned, amorphous mineral deposition (90 ×). **b** Group II, 6 weeks p.f.: massive callus, lamellar bone structure (90 ×)

dardized scanning technique and imaging time, supine position, and equal anatomic positions of both lower extremities. A medium-resolution technetium collimator and scintillation camera were used for the simultaneous imaging and measurement of both extremities.

To permit a quantitative comparison of the distribution of tracer activities in both tibias, we determined the activity of equal-size regions of interest (ROI). In the ROI technique the count rates in the electronically boxed fracture area and the adjacent proximal and distal diaphysis are compared with the count rate in the reference area of the unfractured tibia. This provides a means of quantifying the tracer uptake per unit area and time (Segmüller et al. 1969; Franke et al. 1982).

The activity quotient Q tells us how much tracer uptake is increased in the region of interest compared with the contralateral side. If both tibias are unfractured or if the fracture is scintigraphically healed, the activity quotient $Q = 0.09-1.06$ (Dleditzsch 1980; Koecher and Kiefler 1981). Data were processed with the ERP 1100 computer (Krupp Atlas, Essen).

The activity quotient Q measured in the healthy unfractured tibias of 15 rabbits of the same strain and breed averaged 1.04 (SD 0.04). Scintigraphic

Table 13. ROI activity quotients Q in the fractured/unfractured tibias of both experimental groups at selected times during fracture healing

Days postfracture	Group I Activity quotient			Group II Activity quotient			t value
	n	x̄	SD	n	x̄	SD	
1	11	1.53	0.11				
7	18	3.24	0.43				
14	18	6.44	0.43				
21	8	5.93	0.20	9	6.14	0.20	2.26
28	9	5.36	0.39	9	5.99	0.11	4.66
42	8	4.92	0.43	12	5.72	0.33	4.71
70	9	5.38	0.53	12	3.63	0.12	9.95
126	9	2.65	0.20	10	2.19	0.08	3.41
168	8	1.55	0.39	9	1.06	0.15	3.42
203	5	1.04	0.06				

Table 14. ROI activity quotients in the knee joint: fractured leg/healthy leg at selected times during fracture healing

Days postfracture	Group I Activity quotient			Group II Activity quotient			t value
	n	x̄	SD	n	x̄	SD	
1	11	1.03	0.04				
7	18	1.26	0.09				
14	18	1.39	0.10				
21	8	1.51	0.12	9	1.45	0.10	1.02
28	9	1.22	0.21	9	1.38	0.13	2.05
42	8	1.12	0.04	12	1.20	0.07	2.09
70	9	1.04	0.06	12	1.11	0.06	2.09
126	9	1.02	0.04	10	1.05	0.25	1.04
168	8	1.02	0.04	9	1.00	0.15	0.03

studies were performed in 92 rabbits with tibial fractures (total of 179 scintigrams). The results are summarized in Tables 13 and 14.

Scans of the fractured tibia showed a significant increase in tracer uptake at only 24 h postfracture. Count rates were found to be increased throughout the tibial diaphysis in the initial days following the fracture. The activity quotient in group II was significantly higher on days 21, 28, and 42.

Starting on day 70, markedly lower values of tracer uptake were found in group II compared with group I. By day 168, the fractures in group II were no longer visible on the bone scans. This contrasts with group I, in which scintigrams did not demonstrate bone healing until day 203. By that time the activity quotient had decreased to 1.06 (Fig. 42).

Uptake in the knee joint of the fractured extremity was increased from day 7 to day 42. The maximum ROI activity quotient was measured on day 21. We

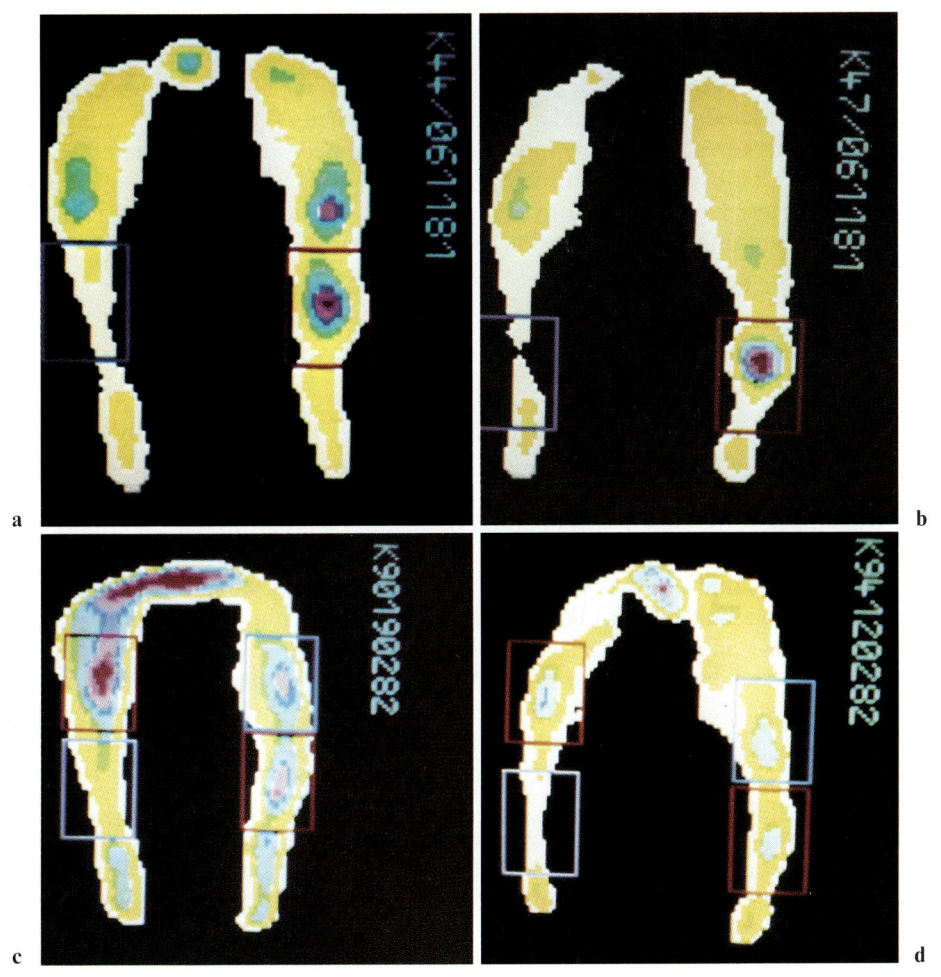

Fig. 42. a Group II, 7 weeks p.f., ROI activity quotient 5.77. **b** Group I, 7 weeks p.f., ROI activity quotient 4.9. **c** Group II, 18 weeks p.f., ROI activity quotient 2.8. **d** Group I, 18 weeks p.f., ROI activity quotient 2.0

found that ^{99m}Tc uptake in the knee joints of the group II animals was not significantly increased on days 28, 42, and 70 compared with group I.

7.5 Angiographic Studies

Angiographic visualization of the intramedullary and callus vessels was performed to determine the number of vessels per unit area and also to determine the direction of vascular branching, which corresponds to the direction of blood flow (Göthmann 1961; Rhinelander 1968, 1974; Dambe 1971; Schweiberer et al. 1973; Trueta 1974; Sturmer and Schuchardt 1980; Eitel et al. 1981).

Following induction of hexobarbital anesthesia, the abdominal aorta was exposed transabdominally, and a 2-mm plastic catheter filled with 0.9% NaCl solution was threaded distally into the aorta and tied into place. Then 80 ml of a 30% Colobaryt/E 153 suspension warmed to 38°C was slowly injected into the arterial system; 8 ml of a 10% formalin solution was added to the suspension to improve its adhesion to the vessel wall.

100 g of Colobaryt consists of:
97.493 g barium sulfate,
 0.007 g oxyphenisatin,
 2.5   g sodium carboxymethylcellulose.

The barium sulfate particles, with a diameter of 1–3 µm, adhere to the vessel wall, become impacted, and slowly occlude the lumen. Vessels less than 0.1 mm in size are not filled. The animals were killed by the rapid intravenous injection of 300 mg hexobarbital. Exarticulation of the tibia was performed 2 h after the Colobaryt injection. The tibia was skinned and fixed for 4 h in 10% formalin. Then the remaining soft tissues were dissected from the bone on the preperiosteal plane, and plain radiographic views were obtained. The bone-callus segment was removed with a saw and decalcified for 14–28 days in a solution of 5% nitric acid and 10% formalin. A polytome was used to obtain sectional radiographs of the decalcified specimens in longitudinal and transverse views. Some of the decalcified specimens were cut into longitudinal or transverse slices 2 mm thick. Finally, magnification radiographs (42 mA, 29 kV, 1/12 s exposure time) were obtained.

On the magnified survey angiograms, a count was made of the barium sulfate-filled vessels that could be identified in an area of periosteal callus measuring 2 cm^2. The direction of the callus vessels and delineation of the nutrient artery were evaluated.

A total of 108 angiograms were made of the lower extremities; 65 had a technical quality that was acceptable for evaluation (Tables 15 and 16, Fig. 43).

Statistical calculations demonstrated an equal number of periosteal callus vessels in both experimental groups. Thus, our findings indicate that the ultrasound treatment of tibial fractures does not significantly influence the number of callus vessels.

7.6 Biochemical Studies

Bone in adult animals consists of approximately 20%–25% water, 45%–65% minerals, 20%–30% inorganic materials, and 15% fat (Schenk and Kolb 1982; Doerr 1974). The inorganic fraction is not only essential to the static and mechanical stability of the bone but plays a vitally important role in maintaining the ionic and electrolyte metabolism of the organism as a

Table 15. Results of angiographic studies

Days p.f.	Nutrient artery	Callus vessels	Course of vessels
1	Divided, interfragmental	None	Distal nutrient artery fills through metaphyseal anastomosis
7	Divided	A few vascular sprouts; 3 vessels/2 cm^2	Obliquely outward and distally from center of callus
14	Divided	Vascular sprouts more numerous, longer, and corkscrew-like; 7 vessels/2 cm^2	Pericortical: transverse and perpendicular; subperiosteal: parallel to bone axis
21	Divided; interfragmental vascular penetration	Mostly in posterior and lateral part of callus, 14 vessels/2 cm^2	Mostly parallel, occasionally perpendicular to bone axis, subperiosteal
28	Incipient anastomosis	Large cross section mostly in distal part of callus, 12 vessels/2 cm^2	Straight and parallel to bone axis, subperiosteal
42	Complete anastomosis on fracture plane	Strong connections with medullary vessels, 8 vessels/2 cm^2	Longitudinal, periosteal
70	Continuity reestablished in diaphyseal region	4 vessels/2 cm^2 periosteal	Longitudinal,
126	Normal medullary arterial system	1 large-caliber callus vessel	Longitudinal

Table 16. Number of vessels in a 2 cm^2 area of fracture callus

Days postfracture	Group I			Group II		
	n	$\bar{x}$	SD	n	$\bar{x}$	SD
7	5	3	2			
14	5	7	3			
21	5	14	5	5	13	5
28	5	12	6	5	11	4
42	5	9	2	5	8	3
70	5	4	2	3	4	2
126	5	1	1	5	1	1

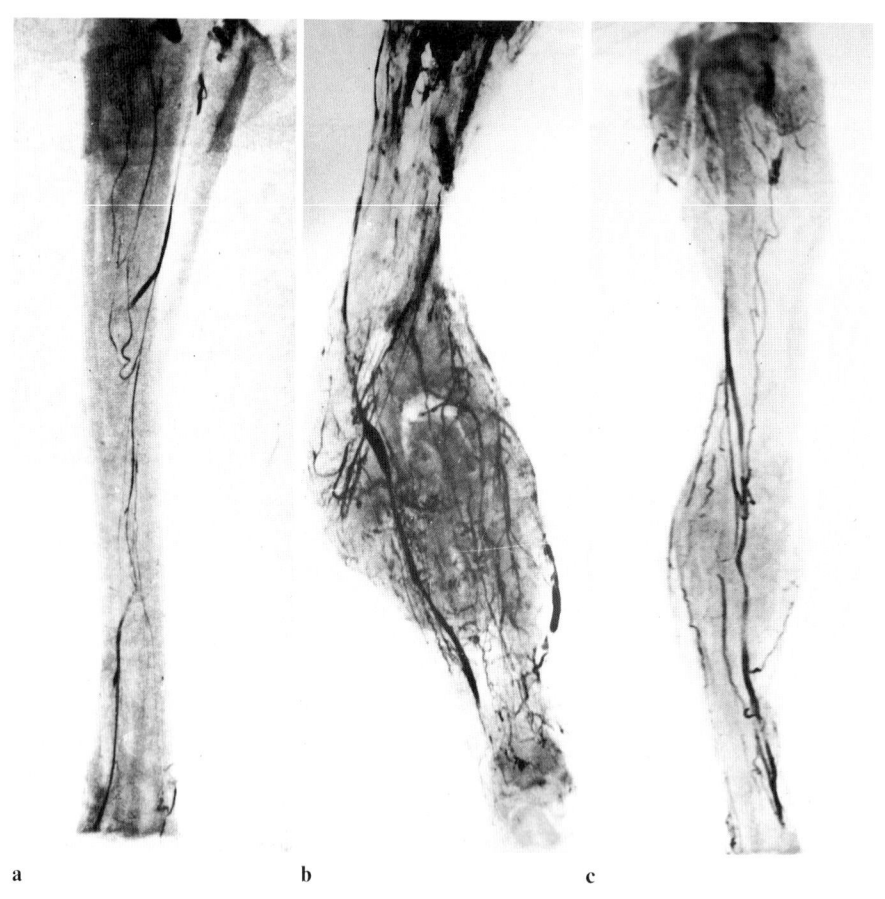

Fig. 43. a Normal course of the opacified nutrient artery in the unfractured tibia. **b** 3 weeks p.f.: Nutrient artery divided, 14 callus vessels/2 cm^2 area of callus, mostly posterior and lateral. No difference between groups I and II. **c** 10 weeks p.f.: Nutrient artery patent, continuity restored; callus vessels less tortuous. No difference between the experimental groups

whole. Bone with deficient mineralization is compromised in its ability to adapt to mechanical loads. During the growth period, minerals are incorporated into bone at a rate exceeding their rate of breakdown. The major inorganic constituents of bone are carbon, sodium, magnesium, phosphorus, potassium, and calcium. Fluorine, chlorine, copper, iron, and zinc are present as trace elements.

An essential step in osteogenesis and fracture healing is the formation of an inorganic solid from the ionic components of the ambient extracellular fluid. The inorganic substances accumulate in mature osteoblasts and mature osteocytes through electrochemical processes (Doerr 1974; Pohl and Goymann 1982). At the cell membrane the ions are drawn into vesicles of lipid composition. The inorganic substances leave the cells as amorphous salts.

Amorphous calcium phosphate is converted to apatite by the action of alkaline phosphates and other mechanisms (Fleisch 1966; Münzenberg 1971). The crystalline fractions grow and bind to collagen fibrils. The crystal axis is directed parallel to the collagen fibrils, giving the structure the properties of a semiconductor. The crystals are situated in and on the fibrils (Robinson 1932). The principal inorganic component of bone is apatite, which is present chiefly as a mixed crystal of carbonate and hydroxyapatite. Other inorganic constituents are fluorapatite and brushite (Münzenberg 1971, 1976), which are also crystalline. These minerals differ greatly in their solubilities.

Determination of Water Content

Following exarticulation of the tibia (removal of the callus or excision of the middle third of the unfractured tibial diaphysis), the wet weight of the callus and bone was determined. The callus and bone were dried for 7 days at 22° C in an environment with 70% atmospheric humidity. Dry weight was subtracted from wet weight to determine the water content of the specimens. The wet weight of the callus was determined for a total of 70 tibial fractures and expressed per g callus.

Water content in 1 g wet bone (tibial diaphysis) measured in 20 bones: $\bar{x} = 0.315$ g (SD 0.082).

The water content of the callus decreases significantly during fracture healing. Our analysis showed that ultrasound exposure had no demonstrable effect on the water content of the tibial fracture callus.

Determination of Alkaline Phosphatase

Robinson showed in 1932 that alkaline phosphatase plays a consistent role in normal osteogenesis. Alkaline phosphatase is formed in preosteoblasts, young osteoblasts, and osteocytoclasts (Doerr 1974; Földes 1976). Its level in the serum and growing callus is elevated during fracture healing by the increased preosteoblastic and osteoblastic activity (Kern et al. 1965; Andersen et al. 1975). Just 2 days after the fracture, alkaline phosphatase can be detected in the periosteum and endosteum. New bone formation commences in the phosphatase-rich callus areas approximately 24 h later, after the enzyme activity has passed its maximum. The function of alkaline phosphatase in fracture healing is the hydrolytic splitting of phosphoric acid monoesters in the blood into phosphate (Rapoport 1977; Lechhorn and Herzog 1977), causing a local increase in the concentration of P ions. Alkaline phosphatase is involved in both maxtrix formation and mineralization. It promotes calcification by increasing the local concentration of P ions, producing a corresponding drain of calcium ions. As the osteoblasts in the bony ground substance are converted to osteocytes, their enzymatic activity progressively declines (Crone-Münzenbrock 1957; Fleisch 1961).

Table 17. Callus alkaline phosphatase content during fracture healing

Days postfracture	Group I [N] [nmol/s · g]			Group II [N] [nmol/s · g]			t value
	n	x̄	SD	n	x̄	SD	
7	13	50.11	1.6				
14	11	57.13	2.6				
21	16	70.01	5.85	16	301.98	24.05	37.56
28	16	90.01	6.05	17	573.31	53.61	33.84
42	14	123,02	5,43	10	118.78	14.54	1.04
70	9	49.61	3.19	12	59.29	10.50	2.78
126	5	39.91	3.28	5	23.58	12.50	2.93
168	5	18.99	2.14	5	13.4	2.80	4.46

The air-dried callus and bone are homogenized in 0.9% NaCl with an electric mixer and stored for 24 h in a refrigerator; the callus solution is manually stirred at frequent intervals. Then the NaCl-callus solution is centrifuged, and the clear supernatant is processed for the determination of alkaline phosphatase.

Alkaline phosphatase was determined by kinetic analysis following a standardized procedure (I DAB 7, D. L.).

The average content of alkaline phosphatase in the bone of the tibial diaphysis measured in 24 healthy bones is $\bar{x} = 11.32 \pm 1.78$ nmol/s.g.

In experimental group II, the content of alkaline phosphatase in the callus on day 21 postfracture is significantly higher than in group I. The highest alkaline phosphatase content is measured on day 28 (Table 17).

On day 42 the alkaline phosphatase is elevated in both experimental groups, and the difference between the groups is not significant. The content on days 126 and 168 postfracture is significantly lower in group II than in group I, reaching the normal value for compact bone on day 168.

pH Measurement

A traumatic tissue injury and subsequent aseptic inflammation are prerequisite conditions for new bone formation (Crone-Münzenbrock 1957; Küntscher 1962). The increased metabolic activity shifts the ionic milieu toward acidity in the initial phase of fracture healing. Crone-Münzenbrock (1957) and Heuwinkel et al. (1980) found that the pH of the callus in the initial days after an experimental fracture was 0.2 lower than the pH of the surrounding soft tissues and bone. Reportedly, a gradual rise in pH is observed following the incorporation of inorganic materials into the callus and the formation of mixed crystals. Küntscher (1962) holds that this shift of pH toward alkalinity creates ideal conditions for increased alkaline phosphatase activity.

Callus pH was measured with the glass electrode of a pH meter (Radiometer, Copenhagen) following a standardized procedure (DAB 7, D. L.). The

Biochemical Studies

Table 18. Callus pH during fracture healing

Days post fracture	Group I			Group II			t value
	n	x̄	SD	n	x̄	SD	
7	10	6.88	0.12				
14	10	6.93	0.17				
21	10	7.11	0.18	10	7.25	0.16	2.09
28	10	7.06	0.15	10	7.20	0.14	2.23
42	10	7.06	0.18	10	7.25	0.13	2.49
70	8	7.03	0.17	9	7.05	0.10	1.06
126	8	7.07	0.16	8	7.11	0.12	0.31
168	9	7.10	0.16	9	7.12	0.11	0.29

Astrup capillary was filled with the clear NaCl-callus solution that was centrifuged for the alkaline phosphatase assay.

The average pH of the healthy compact bone of the tibial diaphysis measured in 40 bones was 7.12 (SD 0.1). Table 18 shows the progression of findings during the course of fracture healing.

In the callus of group II, significant pH shifts toward the alkaline range were measured between days 28 and 42.

Determination of Inorganic Substances

We incinerated the fracture callus in a muffle furnace for 5 days at 550° C. The compact bone of the unfractured tibia also was reduced to ash.

The bone and callus ash were processed as follows for the quantitative analysis of Na, Mg, P, K, Ca, Cu, and Zn:
- The sample was pulverized in the incineration vessel with a glass rod.
- 2 ml HCl (concentrated analytic grade) was added to the sample, which was then heated to complete dissolution of the ash.
- Distilled water was added to the HCl concentrate to make 10 ml, and Na^+, K^+, Cu^{++}, and Zn^{++} were determined.
- 0.1 ml of this solution was diluted with 20 ml distilled water for analysis of Ca^{++}, PO_4^{---}, and Mg^{++}.

The quantities or inorganic substances were analytically determined in parts of mol/l, and the content calculated and expressed per g of dry callus or dry bone.

Sodium, potassium, and calcium were determined by flame photometry using a standardized technique (DAB 7, D. L.) and the Carl Zeiss Model III flame photometer (VEB Zeiss, Jena). Day-to-day deviation was 2%.

Magnesium, zinc, and copper were determined by absorption spectrophotometry following standard procedural guidelines (2. AB, D. L.) and using the Atomsorb unit (LKB Stockholm). Day-to-day deviation was 4%.

Quantitative analysis of phosphorus was done photometrically following a standard method (DAB 7, D. L.).

Sodium content of the compact bone of the unfractured tibial diaphysis measured in 42 bones: $\bar{x} = 0.224$ mmol/g (SD 0.037). Table 19 shows the progression of findings during fracture healing.

The sodium content of the callus in group II does not differ quantitatively from that in group I up to the 70th day postfracture. On days 126 and 168, however, the sodium content is significantly lower in group II.

Magnesium content of the compact bone of the tibial diaphysis measured in 42 bones: $\bar{x} = 0.143$ mmol/g (SD 0.022). The results are summarized in Table 20.

The callus magnesium content in group II is significantly lower on day 28 than in group I, but it is significantly higher on days 42, 70, and 126. In neither group does the value reach the normal value for bone by day 168.

Phosphorus content of the compact bone of the tibial diaphysis measured in 40 bones: $\bar{x} = 3.57$ mmol/g (SD 0.29). The results are summarized in Table 21.

The phosphorus level from day 21 to day 126 is significantly higher in group II than in group I. The content on day 42 approximates that of the compact bone of the unfractured tibia.

Table 19. Callus sodium content during fracture healing

Days post fracture	Group I [nmol/g]			Group II [nmol/g]			t value
	n	$\bar{x}$	SD	n	$\bar{x}$	SD	
7	10	0.06	0.02				
14	10	0.31	0.03				
21	10	0.33	0.02				
28	15	0.25	0.02	10	0.26	0.05	0.21
42	19	0.23	0.02	10	0.23	0.02	0.61
70	10	0.20	0.02	11	0.19	0.02	0.26
126	10	0.29	0.03	10	0.14	0.01	17.01
168	10	0.26	0.02	9	0.10	0.02	16.51

Table 20. Callus magnesium content during fracture healing

Days post fracture	Group I [nmol/g]			Group II [nmol/g]			t value
	n	$\bar{x}$	SD	n	$\bar{x}$	SD	
7	5	0.025	0.018				
14	10	0.079	0.023				
21	10	0.111	0.056	10	0.093	0.010	1.05
28	12	0.063	0.014	12	0.043	0.011	4.04
42	13	0.089	0.027	12	0.106	0.024	2.28
70	12	0.072	0.019	15	0.091	0.070	4.62
126	10	0.075	0.022	13	0.092	0.025	2.28
168	6	0.121	0.017	6	0.123	0.022	0.18

Biochemical Studies

Table 21. Callus phosphorus content during fracture healing

Days post fracture	Group I [nmol/g]			Group II [nmol/g]			t value
	n	x̄	SO	n	x̄	SO	
7	10	0.33	0.25				
14	12	0.83	0.12				
21	8	1.68	0.44	8	2.81	0.23	6.44
28	14	1.57	0.11	14	2.51	0.32	10.39
42	15	2.33	0.67	14	3.38	0.52	5.52
70	15	2.06	0.15	15	3.00	0.11	22.39
126	10	2.34	0.38	15	2.61	0.18	3.2
168	8	3.16	0.59	8	3.38	0.24	0.97

Table 22. Callus potassium content during fracture healing

Days post fracture	Group I [μmol/g]			Group II [μmol/g]			t value
	n	x̄	SD	n	x̄	SD	
7 ˙	10	15.61	1.28				
14	10	31.10	1.33				
21	10	30.10	1.42				
28	11	48.57	2.31	10	35.21	3.12	11.23
42	15	46.57	2.31	19	37.34	3.12	9.56
70	15	30.51	1.48	10	38.34	2.34	10.04
126	10	30.11	2.31	15	28.12	2.56	1.92
168	10	30.17	2.51	10	30.19	3.06	0.08

Potassium content of the compact bone of the tibial diaphysis measured in 15 bones: x̄ = 28.59 mmol/g (SD 0.91). The results are summarized in Table 22.

The potassium content of the callus in experimental group II is significantly below that in group I on days 28 and 42. On day 70 the potassium content is higher in group II than in group I, thereafter returning to the normal value for compact bone.

Calcium content of the compact bone of the tibial diaphysis measured in 45 bones: x̄ = 5.43 mmol/g (SD 0.26). The data are summarized in Table 23.

Starting on day 21 postfracture, the calcium content in group II is significantly elevated in relation to group I: 275% on day 21, 135% on day 28, and 24.5% on day 70. The calcium content reaches that of the compact tibial diaphysis on day 126 in group II, but not until day 168 in group I.

Copper content of the compact bone of the tibial diaphysis measured in 44 bones: x̄ = 56.26 mmol/g (SD 11.47). The data are summarized in Table 24.

Table 23. Callus calcium content during fracture healing

Days post fracture	Group I [nmol/g]			Group II [nmol/g]			t value
	n	$\bar{x}$	SD	n	$\bar{x}$	SD	
7	10	0.38	0.10				
14	10	0.68	0.21				
21	10	0.79	0.22	10	2.98	0.33	17.46
28	12	1.57	0.22	10	4.18	0.23	27.14
42	14	3.37	0.30	15	4.78	0.42	11.03
70	13	3.53	0.47	14	4.80	0.40	9.33
126	10	3.38	0.65	10	5.35	0.36	11.31
168	10	5.58	0.55	10	5.75	0.41	0.91

Table 24. Callus copper content during fracture healing

Days post fracture	Group I [nmol/g]			Group II [nmol/g]			t value
	n	$\bar{x}$	SD	n	$\bar{x}$	SD	
7	5	25.37	12.55				
14	10	44.39	10.54				
21	11	42.89	15.00	13	43.21	11.36	0.06
28	11	41.79	9.04	13	44.01	17.98	0.40
42	16	50.11	13.61	11	51.63	3.80	0.41
70	11	43.75	7.61	15	46.90	5.70	1.60
126	10	41.60	7.82	15	42.56	8.00	0.40
168	8	42.13	3.00	8	38.72	8.03	0.51

Table 25. Callus zinc content during fracture healing

Days post fracture	Group I [μmol/g]			Group II [μmol/g]			t value
	n	$\bar{x}$	SD	n	$\bar{x}$	SD	
7	10	0.80	0.13				
14	10	1.75	0.27				
21	10	2.40	0.21	10	5.88	0.18	7.81
28	10	2.33	0.20	10	5.95	0.17	46.88
42	14	2.49	0.37	14	5.41	0.26	42.48
70	11	2.67	0.33	11	3.22	0.21	26.62
126	10	3.16	0.21	9	3.25	0.31	0.44
168	8	3.32	0.31	8	3.12	0.41	0.98

The copper level is unaffected by ultrasound treatment. The copper content in group I increases until day 14 and remains constant through day 168. It is 20% below the normal value for compact bone.

Zinc content of the compact bone of the tibial diaphysis measured in 43 bones: $\bar{x} = 3.51$ mmol/g (SD 0.78). The results are summarized in Table 22.

In fractures treated with ultrasound, the zinc content of the callus already shows a significant increase by day 21. The increase remains significant until day 70, whereupon the zinc content falls to the normal value for compact bone.

7.7 Total Mineral Analysis

The quantitative measurement of total mineral content is a useful study in all bony injuries that involve the mineral metabolism.

The mineral content of the callus changes during the course of fracture healing. One approach to the quantitative analysis of the total mineral content of callus and bone is the technique inaugurated by Dameron and Sörenson (1963).

We performed the quantitative mineral analysis with the Nordland Cameron Model 178 fully automated bone mineral analyzer (Nordland Instruments, USA). This portable device consists of an analytic section and a computer section. The analytic section consists of a monoenergetic ^{125}I radiation source that emits a collimated beam, and a scintillation detector in the form of a NaI crystal. The callus absorbs the emitted photons in accordance with its mineral content, decreasing the registered count (pulse) rate in the detector. The scintillations are transformed into electrical pulses.

From the integral of the absorption curve, the computer calculates and gives a direct readout of the total mineral content of the sample in g/cm. The major advantage of this device is the direct digital readout of data (Schuster et al. 1969; Börner et al. 1971; Strüter and Rassow 1969; Gordes et al. 1975; Banzer et al. 1976; Kleditzsch 1980; Fengler et al. 1981).

The measurements and results are highly reproducible. Cameron and Sörenson (1963) report a mean error of 2% in determining the bone mineral content and bone thickness. – Comparisons can be made despite variations in bone thickness by computing the "bone index," or the ratio of the measured mineral content and bone diameter in g/cm^2 (Gordes et al. 1975):

$$\text{Bone index} = \frac{\text{mineral content g/cm}}{\text{bone thickness cm}}$$

We determined the bone mineral content and bone thickness at three different sites in the callus, from which all soft tissues had been removed:
- at the largest callus diameter,
- 4 mm above the largest callus diameter,
- 4 mm below the largest callus diameter.

Three measurements were performed at each of these sites. Comparable measurements were performed at three levels in the uninjured tibia:
- center of the tibia,
- 4 mm distal to the center,
- 4 mm proximal to the center.

These distances were used in calculating the mean value of the mineral content of the callus and bone.

Total mineral content of the midshaft tibial diaphysis measured in 22 bones: $\bar{x} = 1.43$ g/cm^2 (SD 0.21). Table 26 shows the progression of findings during fracture healing.

Bone index of the tibial diaphysis measured in 22 bones: $\bar{x} = 0.78$ g/cm^2 (SD 0.19). The results are summarized in Table 27.

The total mineral content of the callus is significantly higher in group II on days 21, 28, 42, and 70 postfracture. Total mineral content is equal in both groups on days 126 and 168.

Table 26. Total mineral content of the callus during fracture healing

Days post fracture	Group I [g/cm^2]			Group II [g/cm^2]			t value
	n	$\bar{x}$	SD	n	$\bar{x}$	SD	
7	10	0.21	0.15				
14	10	0.99	0.17				
21	10	1.20	0.18	10	1.52	0.18	3.32
28	10	1.38	0.12	10	1.92	0.12	8.43
42	10	1.51	0.15	10	1.79	0.11	2.53
70	10	1.66	0.10	10	1.92	0.15	2.88
128	10	1.50	0.15	10	1.51	0.14	0.12
168	10	1.56	0.11	10	1.53	0.13	0.47

Table 27. Bone index during fracture healing

Days post fracture	Group I [g/cm^2]			Group II [g/cm^2]			t value
	n	$\bar{x}$	SD	n	$\bar{x}$	SD	
7	10	0.21	0.07				
14	10	0.35	0.06				
21	10	0.52	0.05	10	0.59	0.13	0.42
28	10	0.61	0.06	10	0.92	0.12	3.15
42	10	0.77	0.11	10	1.26	0.12	2.44
70	10	0.75	0.09	10	0.91	0.09	2.51
126	10	0.73	0.10	10	0.76	0.06	0.08
168	10	0.78	0.12	10	0.75	0.09	0.32

7.8 Sequential Polychrome Labeling

The intravital administration of fluorescent dyes provides a means of studying the progression of growth, remodeling, and healing in callus and bone.

The use of multiple fluorescent markers provides valuable, quantitative information on the time course of fracture healing (Suzuki and Mathews 1966; Perren and Allgöwer 1976; Rahn 1976; Meffert and Kämmerer 1970; Radtke 1975; Stürmer and Schuchardt 1980; Kleditzsch 1980; Schubert 1981).

As indicated by autoradiographic studies with calcium-45, the fluorescent lines that appear in the specimen correspond to sites of calcium deposition (Harris 1960). The actual labeling front affects only the portion of the osteoid seam that is undergoing primary mineralization (Czitober 1963). The process of fluorochrome uptake is analogous in the osteoid of the periosteum, endosteum, and osteon (Meffert and Kämmerer 1970).

The substances used in our sequential labeling experiment are listed in Table 28.

The sterile solutions were prepared and packaged at the pharmaceutical laboratory of Dresden Medical Academy. The fluorochromes were placed in 2% aqueous $NaHCO_3$ solution and dispensed into 10-ml hypodermic ampules. Each 1 ml of the finished sterile solution contained the proper amount of label for 1 kg body weight of the experimental animal.

We injected label subcutaneously on the day of the fracture and at 7/14-day intervals after the fracture. Bone-callus slices 4 mm thick were cut from the fracture area with an oscillating saw and fixed for 24 h in Carnoy's solution. They were dehydrated and degreased in graded alcohols and in xylene. After soaking in a mixture of methylmethacrylate and butylmethacrylate, the bone slices wre embedded using the technique of Wolf and Pompe (1980) as modified by Schubert (1982). A hard section microtome (Model K, Jung, Heidelberg) and hard section knife (HK 1) were used to prepare thin sections of 8–12 μm.

The sections were mounted on gel-coated slides and stained with Giemsa and Masson-Goldner trichrome.

The hard sections were examined under transillumination and evaluated. Photomicrographs were taken with the Ergaval apparatus (VEB Carl Zeiss, Jena) using an exposure time of 60–120. The light source was a high-pressure mercury vapor lamp (HPO 50).

Table 28. Fluorochrome dyes used for sequential labeling

Fluorochrome	[%]	Dose [%]	Ultraviolett fluorescence
Pyrrolidinomethyl-tetracycline	2.5	25	yellow
Alizarine complexone	3	30	red
Xylenol orange	9	90	brownish red
Fluorexone	2	20	green

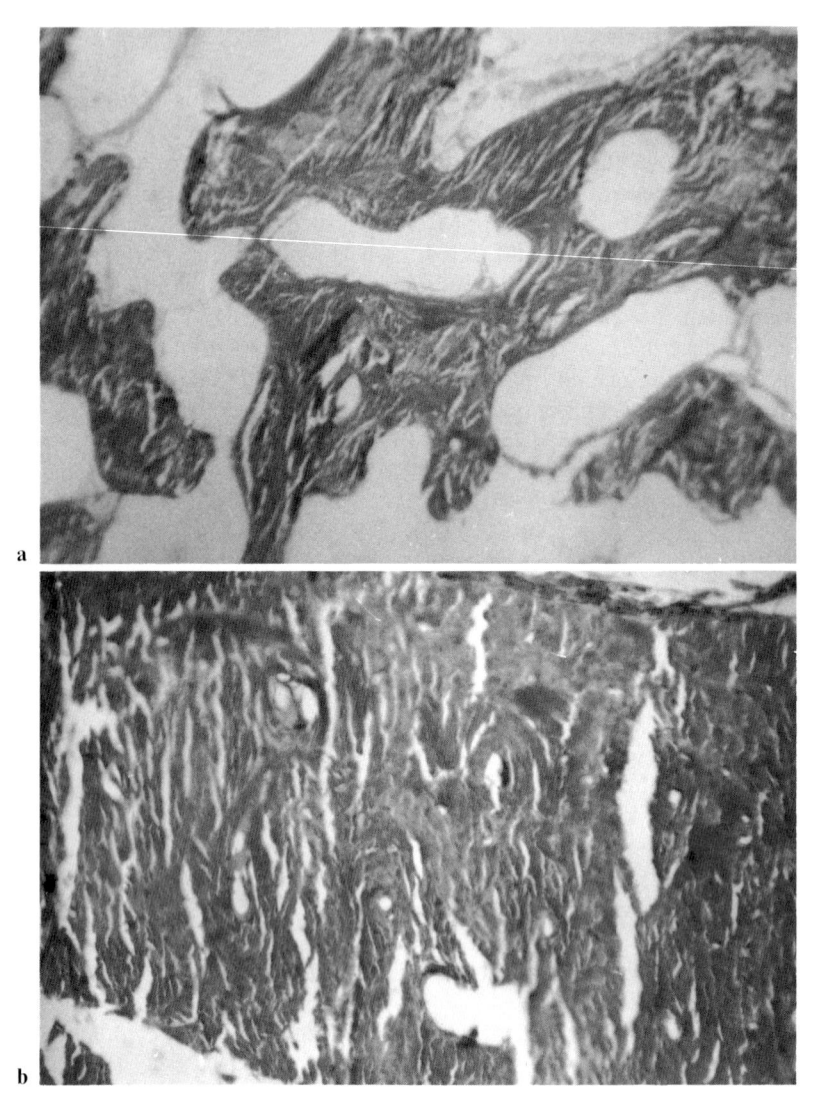

Fig. 44 a,b. Masson-Goldner trichrome stain. **a** Group I, 7 weeks p.f.: spongy callus with narrow osteoid seams. **b** Group II, 7 weeks p.f.: newly formed bone tissue showing normal mineralization

The fluorescent microscopic studies demonstrated increased mineralization of the callus tissue in group II and an accelerated rate of new bone formation. While a spongy callus consisting of fiber bone with narrow osteoid seams was found in group I on day 42, the callus in group II consisted predominantly of newly formed lamellar bone. In these cases there was an early appearance of fiber bone that underwent a rapid conversion to lamellar bone (Fig. 44).

7.9 Temperature Measurements

We performed direct temperature measurements in the live callus, bone, medullary cavity, and rectum using a type Z 8 electric thermometer. The universal electric thermometer (Elektrolab. Ellab, Denmark) operates by the thermocouple principle and is accurate to $\pm 0.1\,°C$ over the range of $16-42\,°C$.

We additionally used the Ellab types R 7 and R 1 standard thermocouple probes for rectal measurements and the type K 3 probe for measuring the temperatures of the callus, compact bone, and medullary cavity.

To rule out heat transfer from the transducer face to adjacent tissues, we measured the temperature on the radiating surface and found the following: Initial temperature: $18\,°C$. At an intensity of $0.2\,W/cm^2$, the temperatures were 17, 16, 16, and $16.5\,°C$ after treatment times of 2, 4, 6, and 8 min; at $0.4\,W/cm^2 - 20, 20.5, 19,$ and $20\,°C$; and at $0.7\,W/cm^2 - 21, 23, 26.5,$ and $28\,°C$ after the same treatment times. We concluded that slight direct heat transfer from the transducer face to the medium is possible only at higher intensities.

The temperature of the healthy tibial compact bone in 10 animals was determined as follows: The skin was incised over the lower third of the extensor surface of the tibia, and a hole was drilled obliquely into the compact bone of the tibial diaphysis. The tip of the Ellab type K 3 standard thermocouple probe was inserted into the drill hole, and the probe connected to the electric thermometer. The lateral extensor surface of the tibia was insonated using circular transducer movements. The temperature change ($°C$) measured at an intensity of $0.05\,W/cm^2$ was $\bar{x} - 0.26$ (SD $- 0.07$); at $0.2\,W/cm^2$, $\bar{x} + 0.49$ (SD $+ 0.22$); at $0.4\,W/cm^2$, $\bar{x} + 0.83$ (SD $+ 0.27$); at $0.7\,W/cm^2$, $\bar{x} + 1.13$ (SD $+ 0.21$); and at $1\,W/cm^2$, $\bar{x} + 1.26$ (SD $+ 0.24$).

The temperature of the compact bone returned to its initial value 240 s after termination of the ultrasound exposure.

The following mean values were measured: rectal temperature in 184 animals $38.4 \pm 2.38\,°C$; medullary cavity temperature in 48 animals $33.55 \pm 2.38\,°C$; rectal-intramedullary temperature difference in 48 animals $4.83 \pm 3.0\,°C$. The temperature differences measured during fracture healing are shown in Table 29.

Table 29. Temperature difference between the rectum and callus during fracture healing

Days post fracture	Group I [°C]			Group II [°C]			t value
	n	$\bar{x}$	SD	n	$\bar{x}$	SD	
7	10	15.61	1.28				
14	10	31.10	1.33				
21	10	30.10	1.42				
28	11	48.57	2.31	10	35.21	3.12	11.23
42	15	46.57	2.31	19	37.34	3.12	9.56
70	15	30.51	1.48	10	38.34	2.34	10.04
126	10	30.11	2.31	15	28.12	2.56	1.92
168	10	30.17	2.51	10	30.19	3.06	0.08

With ultrasound treatment (group II), the callus temperature is significantly higher on days 28 and 42 than in group I. On days 70 and 126 the callus temperature in group I is significantly higher than in group II. The temperature increase in the callus may result from the increase in local metabolic activity.

7.10 Summary of Findings

A control group was used in all the animal experiments, and all findings were tested for statistical significance.

The radiographic examinations demonstrate a markedly better and more rapid onset of callus formation in cases treated with vibration and especially with ultrasound.

Mechanical strength testing shows that maximum fracture load and bending strength are already reached on day 70 postfracture and correspond to the strength values of a healthy unfractured tibia. Without ultrasound treatment, comparable values are not reached until day 126.

Histologic studies demonstrate greater maturity of the callus tissue in cases treated with vibration and ultrasound. Lamellar bone formation commences 5 weeks earlier than in controls not treated with ultrasound. The number of osteoblasts is significantly greater, and by day 28 there are aligned collagen fibers with heavy mineralization. Typical bone structures can be seen by day 42.

The biological activity at the fracture site is especially well documented by bone scintigraphy. Normal activities of uninjured bone can be demonstrated scintigraphically on day 168 in fractures treated with ultrasound – 5 weeks earlier than in the controls. Angiograms demonstrate normal vascularity on day 126, showing no significant difference between experimental groups I and II.

The significantly more rapid pH shift toward alkalinity observed between days 21 and 42 in ultrasound-treated cases is interpreted as signifying the onset of healing. While groups I and II show no differences in the content of water, potassium, sodium, or copper in the fracture callus, the calcium and magnesium contents are significantly increased in group II. Higher levels of alkaline phosphatase, phosphorus, and zinc also are measured as an expression of increased mineralization.

Mineralization in group II is complete by day 70 postfracture. The total mineral contents in both groups do not equalize until day 126, a finding that is supported by our fluorescent microscopic studies.

Temperature measurements indicate a temperature rise of up to 1 °C in the fracture area as an expression of increased metabolic activity. This temperature is significantly lower in group II on day 70, indicating a return to normal metabolic function.

Impedance measurements demonstrate a significantly higher electrical conductivity in group II consistent with a normalization of tissues at the fracture site.

Appendix on Instrumentation

The animal experiments as well as our clinical treatments are performed with instruments that are commercially available and are widely used in physiotherapy departments and medical practices.

High-Frequency Instruments

The TuR US 6-1 ultrasound therapy instrument (its technical characteristics, representative of current high-frequency therapy instruments, are listed in Table 30) is a table-top unit of plug-in design. All switches and indicators on the control panel are easy to see and use (Fig. 45). The fuse holders are on the back of the unit, where the power cord and transducer cords are also located. Holders for the transducers are mounted on the sides of the unit. The transduc-

Table 30. Technical characteristics of the US 6-1 ultrasound therapy instrument

Power source:	Grounded AC outlet
Power supply frequency:	50 Hz to 60 Hz
Power supply voltage:	127 V or 220 V
Supply voltage tolerance:	$\pm 10\%$
Maximum current consumption:	1.2 A at 127 V 0.7 A at 220 V
Ultrasound frequency:	800 kHz $\pm 5\%$
Operating modes:	Continuous Pulsed (sinusoidal half wave, pulse repetition frequency 50 Hz)
Radiating area:	Large transducer: 6.4 cm^2 Small transducer: 1.4 cm^2
Intensity control:	Continuous from 0.05 to 2 W/cm^2 in continuous mode Continuous from 0.05 to 0.75 W/cm^2 in pulsed mode
Intensity meter:	Direct readout in W/cm^2
Coupling fault indicator:	Visual with automatic power cutoff and timer shutoff in continuous-mode operation
Treatment timer:	0–30 min with automatic power cutoff, gives audible signal when set treatment time is elapsed; measures effective treatment time in continuous-mode operation

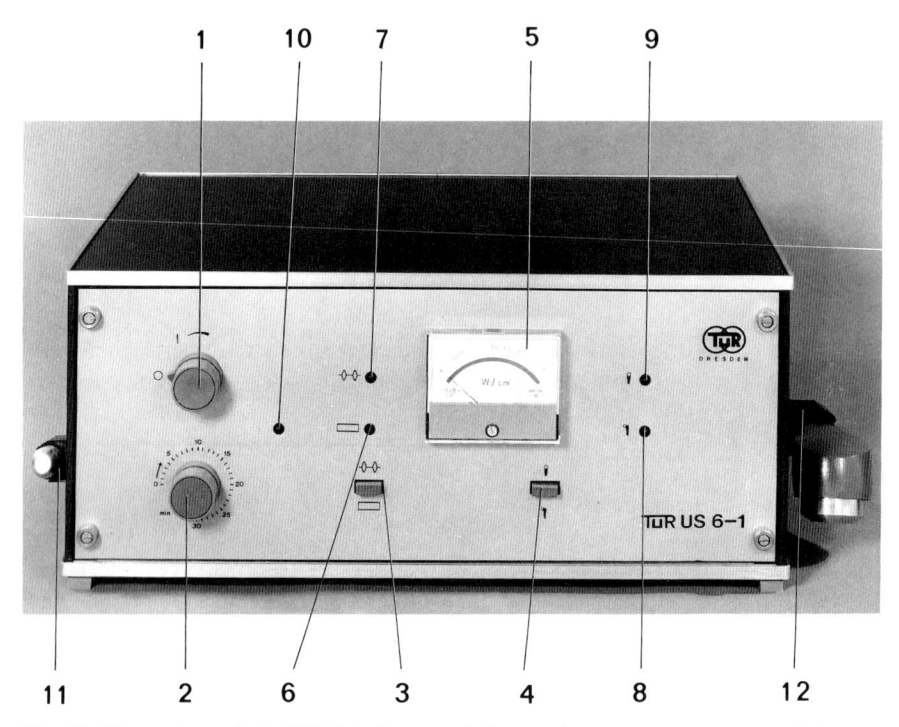

Fig. 45. Front view of the US 6-1 ultrasound therapy instrument. *1* Power switch, also controls intensity; *2* treatment timer; *3* mode selector; *4* transducer selector; *5* intensity meter; *6, 7* mode indicator lights for the selected transducer (*8, 9*); *10* coupling error light for continuous mode; *11* holder for small transducer; *12* holder for large transducer

er, or soundhead, consists of the applicator sleeve, the metal radiating plate (transducer face), and the handle, into which the connecting cord is inserted. The transducers are watertight and suitable for underwater use. The ultrasound level displayed on the intensity meter is valid for sound transmission in water, whose acoustic data are largely equivalent to those of human tissue. Each soundhead contains a ceramic barium titanate transducer that is bonded to the metal radiating plate.

The high-frequency electrical voltage delivered to the transducer through the cord generates mechanical vibrations of equal frequency (reverse piezoelectric effect) which are transmitted to the radiating plate and from there into the coupling medium or patient. These vibrations, and thus the transmitted ultrasound intensity, are greatest when the resonant frequency of the transducer matches that of the high-frequency electrical voltage. The frequency of the transducer must be tuned, therefore; this is done once at the factory. A constant operating frequency is automatically maintained. The power output of the unit, and thus the ultrasound intensity, is controlled by adjusting the control grid voltage of the transmission tube. The TuR US 6-1 can operate in either of two modes. In the □□ rectangle mode the unit produces continuous ultrasound at an intensity of 0.05 to 2 W/cm^2; in the -◊-◊- diamond mode it produces pulsed ultrasound in the form of sinusoidal half waves. The duty factor (ratio of pulse duration to period) is 1:2 with a period of 20 ms.

The intensity in this mode ranges from 0.05 to 0.75 W/cm^2. Power output is measured with a microammeter calibrated in W/cm^2, whose deflection is proportional to the HF voltage applied to the transducer.

The coupling fault indicator functions only in the continuous mode. It is activated when less than 50% of the area of the transducer face is in acoustic contact with the patient. If this occurs, the power is lowered to a minimum, the timer is stopped, and the signal light comes on. The intensity meter is switched off. Once good acoustic contact has been reestablished, the light goes off, the previous power setting is restored, and the timer continues to run.

The unit should always be connected to a grounded power outlet (127 V or 200 V AC, 50–60 Hz). It is designed for operation at 220 V, 50–60 cycles.

After the instrument is switched on, the mode and transducer switches are set to select the desired operating mode (switch 3) and transducer (switch 4). These settings are confirmed by lights on the control panel. After 5 min the instrument is ready for use. The timer is set to the desired treatment time, the transducer is coupled to the patient, and the intensity control is turned to the right to the required setting, which is displayed on the intensity meter.

The treatment is continued until the timer runs out, the signal sounds, and the power is shut off.

The intensity should always be turned down when the unit is switched from one operating mode to the other.

If the coupling error light comes on during continuous-mode operation, the transducer position should be adjusted until the light goes off, confirming restoration of good acoustic contact.

When treatment is completed, the audible signal can be switched off by turning the timer knob to 25–30 min. The intensity control is turned back to "I," and the transducer is returned to its holder. After the next patient has been prepared, the timer is set to the desired time, the transducer is coupled to the patient, the intensity level is set, and the next treatment is started. The instrument is not switched off between multiple consecutive treatments; the intensity is merely turned down.

When all treatments have been completed, the intensity (power) switch is turned to the left until the unit shuts off (indicator lights go out). It is also good practice to remove the plug from the power outlet.

The transducers and cords should be handled with care. A transducer should never be moved by pulling on the soundhead or cord. Twisting and kinking of the cords should be avoided.

It is important to avoid damage to the radiating surface (face) of the transducer, because the slightest damage will decrease the acoustic output.

The soundhead should be lightly greased for immersion treatment. Care is taken that the transducer head is screwed firmly into the applicator sleeve so that water will not seep into the interior of the soundhead. If this occurs, the water should be removed by unscrewing the applicator sleeve. When the soundhead is reassembled, the screw threads should be greased with vaseline or silicone. For cleaning and disinfection of the soundheads, agents should be used that are not corrosive to aluminum. Soundheads should never be heat-sterilized. Also, coupling media and disinfectants should be kept away from the transducer cord. For water immersion treatment, the short transducer handle should be replaced by the long handle.

A careful and precise insonation technique is crucial to success. During treatment, a suitable coupling medium (oil or water) must be present between the transducer face and the body part to be treated. An air layer as thin as 0.1 mm can block ultrasound transmission from the transducer to the patient. The ultrasound can be applied:
- by stroking movements of the transducer,
- by circular movements of the transducer,
- with a stationary transducer (static insonation).

The transducer may be directly coupled to the patient through a thin layer of coupling gel or oil, which is liberally applied to the skin, or a standoff technique may be used in which sound is transmitted to the skin over a distance of about 1–2 cm through a thicker coupling layer. This requires immersion in a water bath using a large or small basin, depending on the body part that is to be treated. The basin is filled with degassed water, and the body part is immersed. The water can be degassed by boiling. Air bubbles adhering to the skin should be wiped off. Immersion treatments are performed with the large transducer mounted on the long handle.

Another instrument, which permits the use of continuous or pulsed ultrasound as well as the application of electric current, is the Rehaphon M 200, manufactured by the Dr. Born company (Fig. 46).

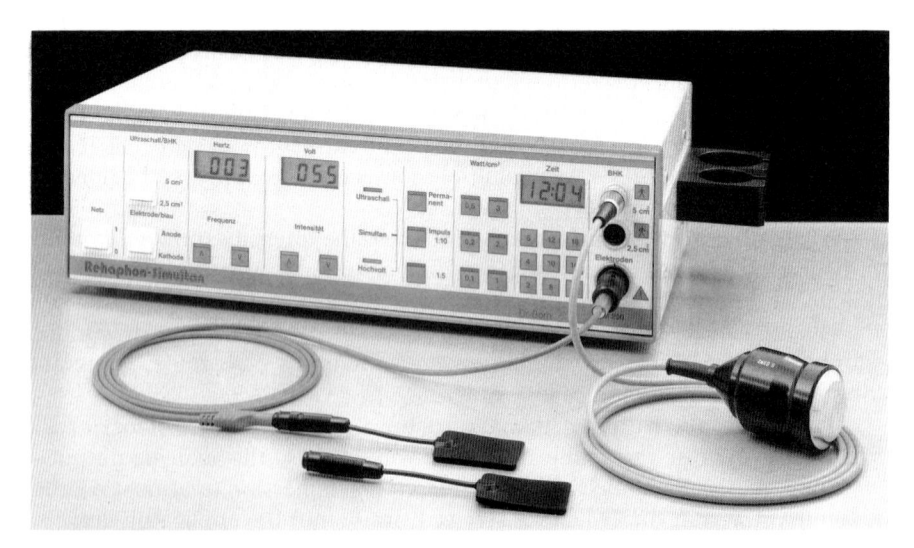

Fig. 46. Example of a therapy instrument that can provide continuous/pulsed ultrasound or electrical stimulation (Rehaphon M 200, Dr. Born Co., Frankfurt)

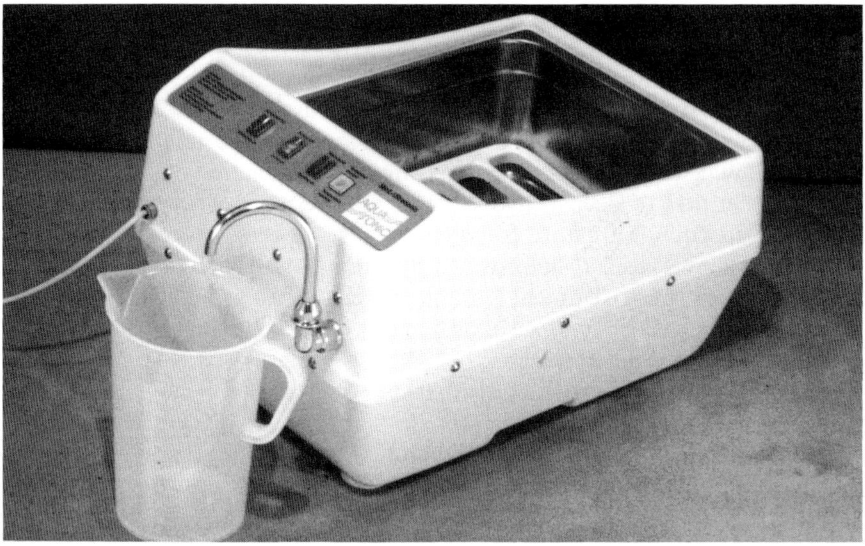

High-Frequency Instruments

Fig. 47. Aqua-Sonic Model 2002 low-frequency immersion therapy unit, for treatment of the foot

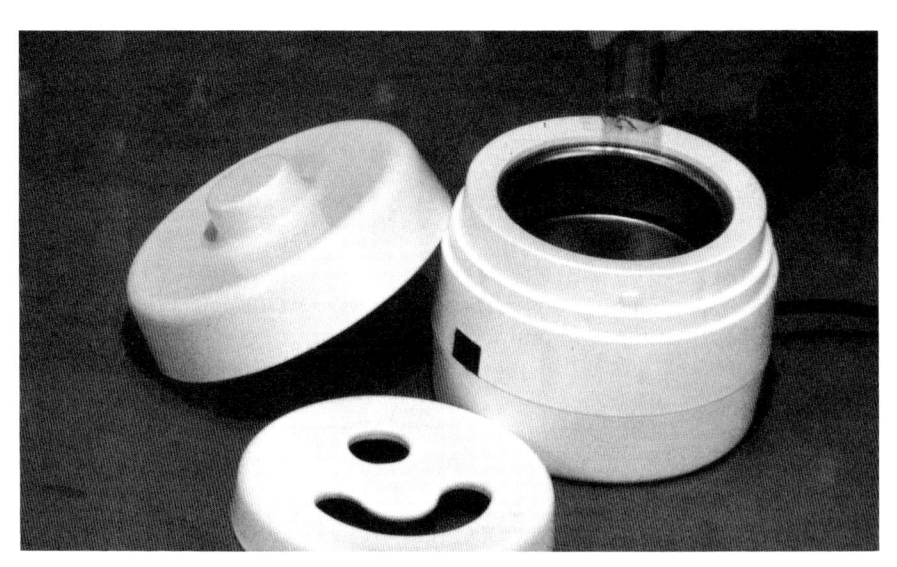

Fig. 48. Aqua-Sonic Model 1002 low-frequency immersion therapy unit, for treatment of the hand

Low-Frequency Instruments

The only manufacturer of low-frequency ultrasound therapy units is Aqua-Sonic (7540 Neuenbürg, FRG). This therapy is distinguished by a very long ultrasound wave, like that used in stomatology for the removal of dental calculus. Tissue damage is ruled out, as only a small fraction of the ultrasound energy penetrates to deeper layers. Thus, low-frequency instruments can be especially useful for treating fractures in cases where there are coexisting ulcerations and a need to improve local blood flow. There is no danger of coupling errors, since treatment is administered in a water bath. The following actions of low-frequency ultrasound have been documented in hundreds of treatment sessions:
- improvement of blood flow (temperature increase);
- increased oxygen delivery (pO_2);
- removal of wound deposits and necrotic debris;
- liquidation of microorganisms (bacteria and fungi are destroyed by cavitation).

Instruments:
a) Model 2002, foot basin with 7-liter capacity, drained by a water pump. Frequency 40 kHz; intensity is controlled by adjusting the current from 0 to 75 W. The unit is automatically switched off by a time relay. Power source 200 V (Fig. 47).
b) Model 2001, hand basin with 200-ml capacity. A lid with finger openings fits on top of the basin. Technical parameters are the same as for Model 2002 (Fig. 48).

Safety Aspects

For safety reasons the user should scrupulously follow the manufacturer's instructions, including any tips or guidelines that are offered. The following rules and considerations are important in daily practice:
- Only a properly grounded power outlet should be used. This should be checked by an electrician.
- The therapist must be familiar with the use and operation of the instrument. The instrument should be used only if it is in proper working condition.
- The appropriate supervisor or service facility should be notified at once if the instrument suffers any damage or operational defect, or if the indicators (lights, dials) are not working.
- The unit should be serviced only by qualified personnel at the place of manufacture.
- If the basin for water immersion treatment has a metal drainpipe that is connected to the sewage system, it is a good precaution to have an electrician connect the grounding conductor of the power outlet to the water

pipes, which in turn are electrically connected to the drainpipe of the therapy unit. This is not essential, however.
- For water immersion treatment, the factory supplies a long-handled transducer holder so that the therapist will not come in contact with the ultrasound vibrations in the water. The short-handled transducer holder also may be immersed in water. If immersion of the therapist's hand cannot be avoided, protective gloves can be worn.
- The accuracy of the intensity meter (W/cm^2) should be checked at designated intervals with an ultrasound power testing instrument.

References

Anderson HC, Russel C, Sagdera SW (1975) Calcification of rachitic rat cartilage in vitro by extracellular matrix vesicles. Am J Pathol 79:237–245

Arnold G, Kokemohr M (1973) Funktionelle Eigenschaften von Röhrenknochen unter axialer Belastung. Z Exp Chir u Chir Forsch 6:68–75

Aro H, Eerola E, Aho AJ (1981) Healing of experimental fractures in the denervated limbs of the rat. Clin Orthop 155:211–216

Baldes EJ, Herrick JF, Stroebel CF (1958) Biologic effects of ultrasound. Am J Phys Med 37:111–117

Banzer D. Klemm T, Schneider U (1976) Der Mineralgehalt des wachsenden Knochens. Dtsch Med Wochenschr 101:1794–1797

Basset A, Pawluk R (1964) Effects of electricity on bone in vivo. Nature 14:652–654

Basset CAL (1965) Electrical effects in bone. Sci Am 18:213–215

Basset CAL, Pawluk RJ (1979) Noninvasive methods for stimulating osteogenesis. J Biomed Mater Res 9:371–374

Basset CAL (1962) Current concepts of bone formation. J Bone Joint Surg [Am] 44:1217–1244

Bauer K, Kinzel L, Wolter D (1974) Untersuchungen zur Knochenbruchheilung unter Einfluß von elektrischem Gleichstrom. Z Orthop 112:402–407

Baumann A, Presch H (1950) Histologische Veränderungen nach Ultraschalleinwirkung auf gesundes Tiergewebe. Strahlentherapie 81:143

Becker DO, Bachmann CH (1965) Bioelectric effects in tissues. In: Letters to the Editor. Clin Orthop 43:251–254

Becker W, Dreyer J, Georgi P (1974) Wert der Szintigraphie bei Frakturen und Pseudarthrosen. Hefte Unfallheilkd 37:242–247

Bessler W (1970) Bedeutung szintigraphischer Untersuchungen nach Frakturen- und Knochenoperationen. Langenbecks Arch Chir 327:146–159

Bethge FJ (1976) Biochemische Beeinflussung der Knochenbruchheilung. Nova Acta Leopoldina 44:145–154

Blietz R (1976) Die biologische Reaktion der Knochen-Cortikalis auf definierte mechanische Spannung als piezoelektrisches Verhalten interpretiert. Nova Acta Leopoldina 44:95–99

Böhme G, Kaltofen S, Petzold D (1981) Entwicklung polarographischer Meßsysteme zur transkutanen extrakorporalen und Gewebs pO_2-Bestimmung. Dtsch Gesundh-Wesen 36:675–680

Börner W, Moll E, Rauli E, Heier G (1971) Ein empfindliches Meßverfahren zur radiologischen Bestimmung der Mineralsalzdichte in Spongiosa und Kompakta der Fingerknochen. Z Orthop 108:503–507

Brandt G (1974) Spurenelementgehalt in Leber, Knochen und Ovar. Z Gerontol 8:28–33

Busnel R, Chauhard RP, Mazone H (1954) Recherches électrophysiologiques sur les conditions d'efficacité des ultra-sons utilisés en thérapeutique. J Radiol 35:847

Buzdanov NV, Kostanko MS, Kuzovlev OP, Mschukaeva V, Rahmillivich LS, Mosipov N (1977) The effect of electrostimulation on the osteogenesis and medullary hemopoesis. Ortop Travmatol Protez 7:31–33

Callies R (1978) Differenzierte Ultraschalltherapie und ihr Einsatz in der Sportmedizin. Med Sport 18:286–291

Callies R, Danz J, Smolenski U (1983) Dosierungsstrategie einer Ultraschalltherapie. Z Physiother 35:259–264
Cameron JR, Sörenson J (1963) Measurement of bone mineral in vivo, an improved method. Science 142:230–232
Carstensen EL, Müller MW, Linke CA (1974) Biological effects of ultrasound. J Biophys Biochem Cytol 2:173–177
Chivers RC (1981) Tissue characterization, Ultrasound. Med Biol 7:1–30
Cieszynski T (1973) Die klinischen Aspekte der bioelektrischen Polarisation. Chirurg 44:559–562
Cieszynski T, Idzikowski A, Goymann V (1982) Biophysikalische Aspekte des Knochenwachstums und der Frakturheilung. Z Orthop 120:527–531
Coakley WT (1978) Biophysical effect of ultrasound at therapeutic intensities. Physiotherapy 64:166–170
Conradi E, Schuldes H, Fritze U, Winterfeld H-J (1983) Zum gegenwärtigen Stand der Therapie mit Impulsultraschall. Z Physiother 35:85–93
Conradi E, Fritze U, Hoffmann B (1983) Untersuchungen zur Verteilung der Wärmeenergie in verschiedenen Gewebsschichten beim Schwein nach Ultraschalltherapie im Gleich- und Impulsbetrieb. Z Physiother 35:271–280
Creutzig H, Gerd KG, Gerdts C, Creutzig A (1977) Vergleichende Untersuchungen mit osteotropen Radionukliden. Dynamik der Anreicherung in normalen und pathologisch veränderten Knochen. Fortschr Röntgenstr 126:258–262
Crone-Münzebrock A (1957) Tierexperimentelle Untersuchungen zur Kallusbildung unter hormonalen Einflüssen mit Berücksichtigung des Verhaltens von Grundsubstanz und Phosphatase. Bruns Beitr Klin Chir 195:1–45, 185–205
Currey JD (1964) Three analogies to explain the mechanical properties of bone. J Biochem 2:1–10
Czitober H (1963) Über eine fluoreszenzmikroskopische Methode zum möglichen Nachweis anaboler Wirkungen am Knochengewebe. Berlin, Anabolika Kolloquium der Fa. Schering KG
Dambe LT (1971) Revaskularisation der Diaphyse langer Röhrenknochen nach Fraktur und Osteosynthese. Med. Dissertation, Universität Saarland
Danz J, Geske G (1977) Zur Frage der Ultraschallreflexion bei Verwendung verschiedener Koppelsubstanzen. Physiother 99:201–207
Danz J, Callies R (1978) Thermometrische Untersuchungen bei unterschiedlichen Ultraschallintensitäten. Z Physiother 30:335–340
Demeter G, Matyas I (1978) Mikroskopisch vergleichend anatomische Studien an Röhrenknochen mit besonderer Berücksichtigung auf die Unterschiede menschlicher und tierischer Knochen. Z Anat 87:45–99
Doerr W (1974) Organpathologie, Band III. Thieme, Stuttgart
Dyson M (1982) Non-thermal cellular effects of ultrasound. Br J Cancer 45:165–171
Eger W (1963) Kalziumnachweis und Mineralisation des Knochengewebes. Verh Dtsch Ges Pathol 47:54–69
Ehler E, Lösche H (1970) Die menschliche Tibia unter Biegebelastung. Beitr Orthop Traumatol 17:291–304
Eitel F, Seiler H, Schweiberer L (1981) Vergleichende morphologische Untersuchungen zur Übertragbarkeit tierexperimenteller Ergebnisse auf den Regenerationsprozeß des menschlichen Röhrenknochens. I. Mitteilung: Untersuchungsmethode. II. Mitteilung: Untersuchungsergebnisse. Z Unfallheilkd 84:250–254, 255–264
Enzler MA, Waelchli-Suter C, Perren SM (1980) Prophylaxe der Pseudarthrose durch magnetische Stimulation. Z Unfallheilkd 83:188–194
Fengler F, Franke J, Runge H, Kramer B (1981) Peripherer Knochenmineralgehalt bestimmt mittels Photonenabsorptionsmessungen an einer Bevölkerungsgruppe des Bezirkes Halle. Beitr Orthop Traumatol 28:408–417
Fleisch H (1961) Neue Gesichtspunkte der Kalkablagerung. Schweiz Med Wochenschr 91:858–861

References

Fleisch H (1966) Physiologie und Biochemie der Knochenbildung. Klin Wochenschr 11:360–363

Földes J (1976) Die Bedeutung von Phosphatestern in der Knochenbildung. Nova Acta Leopoldina 44:155–158

Friedenberg ZB, Zemsky LM, Pollis RP, Brighton CT (1974) The response of nontraumatized bone to direct current. J Bone Joint Surg [Am] 56:1023

Friedenberg MD, Kohanin M (1968) The effect of direct current on bone. Surg Gynecol Obstet 127:97–102

Franke W-G, Kleditzsch J, Beer L, Woller P, Hellinger J (1982) Knochenszintigraphie zur Verlaufskontrolle der Frakturheilung unter Elektrostimulation – tierexperimentelle Untersuchungen. Nucl Compact 13:142–146

Fritze U (1982) Vergleichende Untersuchungen der thermischen Wirkung bei Applikation von impulsiertem und kontinuierlichem Ultraschall. Med. Dissertation, Universität Berlin

Fukuda E, Yasuda I (1957) On the piezoelectric effect of bone. J Phys Soc Jap 12:1158–1161

Fukuda E, Yasuda I (1964) Piezoelectric effects in collagens. J Appl Phys Japan 3:117–122

Gerlanc M, Haddad D, Hyatt GW, Langloh J, Hilaire PS (1975) Ultrasonic study of normal and fractured bone. Clin Orthop 111:175–180

Gordes W, Kossyk W, Bödefeld P (1975) Versuche zur Kalksalzdichtebestimmung an der osteotomierten und stabilisierten Tibia des Kaninchens. Arch Orthop Unfallchir 81:125–147

Göthmann L (1961) Vascular reactions in experimental fractures. Acta Chir Scand 284:1–34

Haefely E, Kleditzsch J, Güttler P (1982) Möglichkeiten der Beeinflussung der Knochenbruchheilung durch elektrische Ströme. Dtsch Gesundh-Wesen 37:629–633

Harris WH (1960) A microscopic method of determining bone growth. Nature 108:38–43

Heimann D, Keller R, Schlachetzki J (1973) Über das Verhalten der alkalischen Serumphosphatase während Frakturheilung. Monatsschr Unfallheilk 76:168–174

Heuwinkel R, Schneider HM, Störkel S (1980) Der Gewebe-pH als Stimulans desmaler Knochenneubildung. Z Unfallheilkd 83:577–585

Hoffmann H, Müller P, Heiner H, Thieme V (1982) Histologische Untersuchungen zur Frakturheilung nach Druckplattenosteosynthese am Hundeunterkiefer. Stomatol Ogiia [Mosk] 32:567–573

Jäger M, Gördes W (1976) Bruchfestigkeit bei konservativ und operativ behandelten Osteotomien der Kaninchentibia. Z Unfallheilkd 79:193–201

Kern E, Weller S, Loch H, Gruber R (1965) Untersuchungen zum Verhalten der alkalischen Serumphosphatase während der Frakturheilung. Monatsschr Unfallheilkd Vers Med 68:313–315

Kihn J (1956) Sauerstoffdiffusion durch die Haut nach verschiedenen physikalischen Einwirkungen. Arch Phys Ther 8:103

Kirchhoff G, Six H (1979) Digitale Registrierung und rationelle Auswertung von Meßdaten der akustischen Emission. Feingerätetechnik 28:163–165

Kleditzsch J (1980) Die Knochenheilung im Tierexperiment unter Einfluß von bipolaren Rechteckimpulsfolgen und Interferenzstrom. Promotion B, Med. Akademie Dresden

Klug W (1983) Tierexperimentelle Untersuchungen über die Wirkung des Ultraschalls auf Knochenbruchheilung, Kallusgewebe und paraklinische Aspekte. Habilitationsschrift, Med Akademie Dresden

Klug W, Knoch H-G (1986) Durch biophysikalische Untersuchungen Quantifizierung der Knochenbruchheilung nach Ultraschallstimulation von distalen Radiusfrakturen. Beitr Orthop Traumatol 33:384–391

Klug W, Knoch H-G (1987) Aktivierung der Knochenbruchheilung durch Ultraschall. Z Physiother 39:91–98

Knoch H-G (1966) Der Einfluß von Nieder- und Hochfrequenzschwingungen – speziell Ultraschall – auf die Kallusbildung. Habilitationsschrift, Med. Akademie Dresden

Knoch H-G (1967) Konservative Behandlungsmöglichkeiten durch Ultraschall bei verzögerter Kallusbildung. Beitr Orthop Traumatol 14:720–726

Knoch H-G (1967) Beiträge zur Wirkungsweise der Ultraschallenergie. Strahlentherapie 134:629-634
Knoch H-G, Dominok GW, Schramm H (1971) Ultraschallfernwirkung auf das Kallusgewebe. Z Exp Chir Chir Forsch 3:248-250
Knoch H-G, Knauth K (1981) Therapie mit Ultraschall, 3. Aufl. VEB Gustav Fischer, Jena
Knoch H-G, Klug W (1988) Schnellere Knochenbruchheilung durch Ultraschall. Der Allgemeinarzt 7:502-511
Knoch H-G (1989) Der niederfrequente Ultraschall – Übersicht. Z Physiother 41 (im Druck)
Koecher W, Kiefler J (1981) Der Einfluß der Sympathektomie auf die Knochendurchblutung. Zentralbl Chir 106:862-872
Kohlrausch W (1955) Reflexionsmassage in Muskulatur und Bindegewebe. Thieme, Stuttgart
Kraus W (1974) Zur Biophysik der Knochenbruch- und Wundbehandlung durch funktionelle elektrische und magnetische Potentiale. Langenbecks Arch Chir 337:625-630
Kraus W (1978) Therapie des Knochens und des Knorpels mit schwacher, langsamschwingender elektromagnetischer Energie. Med Orthop Technik 98:33-43
Küntscher G (1962) Das Kallusproblem. Schattauer, Stuttgart
Kurz W (1981) Verletzung der Epiphysenfuge und Knochenwachstum. Z Exp Chir Chir Forsch 14:98-106
Lechhorn E, Herzog A (1977) Ist die Serum-Aktivität der alkalischen Phosphatase als Hilfsmittel für die HD Diagnose geeignet? Kleintierpraxis 20:145-177
Lehmann J, Delateur B, Warren CG (1967) Healing produced by ultrasound in bone and soft tissue. Arch Phys Med 48:397-401
Lechner F (1976) Klinische Ergebnisse der elektrodynamischen Knochenbruchheilung. Nova Acta Leopoldina 223:127-142
Meffert O, Kämmerer H (1970) Das Fluoreszenzverhalten von Tetracyclindepots in Knochen und Zähnen. Langenbecks Arch Chir 328:254-258
Milachowski K, Moschinski D, Stawinoga B (1981) Das Verhalten der Spurenelemente Kupfer und Zink bei der Knochenbruchheilung des Kaninchens. Z Unfallheilkd 84:168-174
Minta P (1973) Die Rolle des maximalen Achsendrucks in der Fixierung und Heilung der Schaftbrüche der langen Röhrenknochen. Z Exp Chir 6:115-125
Müller Th, Wehner W (1979) Gegenwärtiger Stand der Ultraschallsynthese in der Unfallchirurgie. Beitr Orthop Traumatol 26:570-576
Münzenberg KJ (1971) Die Calzifikation bei der Knochenbildung. Arch Orthop Unfallchir 71:41-54
Münzenberg KJ, Rössler H (1976) Physikalische Veränderungen des Kallusgewebes durch Knochenmineraleinlagerung. Nova Acta Leopoldina 223:257-262
Nödl F (1949) Zur Frage der selektiven Wirkung des Ultraschalls auf die Basaliomzelle. Strahlentherapie 79:289
Otto W (1955) Ultraschalltherapie von Sportverletzungen. Dtsch Gesundheitswesen 10:770
Pauwels F (1972) Eine neue Therapie über den Einfluß mechanischer Reize auf die Differenzierung der Stützgewebe. Z Anat Entwickl-Gesch 121:478-483
Pawluk RJ, Basset CAL (1970) Elektromechanical factors in healing cortical bone defects. Calcif Tissue Int 4:120-121
Perren M, Allgöwer M (1976) Biomechanik der Frakturheilung nach Osteosynthese. Nova Acta Leopoldina 44:61-84
Perren M, Cordey J (1977) Die Gewebsdifferenzierung in der Frakturheilung. Unfallheilkd 80:161-164
Pohl JP, Goymann V (1982) Die elektrochemischen Grundprinzipien des Knochenwachstums und deren Beeinflußbarkeit. Z Orthop 120:439-440
Poljakow WA, Wolkow SM (1972) Die Vereinigung von Knochen mit Hilfe von Ultraschall. Chirurgija 47:10-17
Pospišilova J (1973) Biologische Veränderungen im Granulationsgewebe nach Ultraschallwirkung. Wiss. Z. Humboldt-Universität Berlin 22:382-385

Quasdorf O, Jahn K (1976) Festigkeitsprüfung am Kallus. Nova Acta Leopoldina 223:263–265
Radtke G (1975) Tierexperimentelle Studien über den Einfluß antibiotischer Substanzen, insbesondere der Tetrazykline, auf qualitative Bioparameter der Zahnhartgewebe. Promotion B, Med. Akademie Dresden
Rahn BA (1976) Die polychrome Sequenzmarkierung des Knochens. Nova Acta Leopoldina 44:249–255
Rapoport SM (1977) Medizinische Biochemie 3. Aufl, Verlag Volk und Gesundheit, Berlin
Rautenberg R (1973) Rasterelektronenmikroskopische Untersuchungen des sogenannten Elektrokallus an der Anode und an der Kathode im Tierversuch. Z Orthop 111:620–630
Rhinelander FW (1968) The normal microcirculation of the diaphyseal cortex and its response to fracture. J Bone Joint Surg [Am] A50:748–757
Rhinelander FW (1974) Tibial blood supply in relation to fracture healing. Clin Orthop 105:34–41
Ritter G, Grünert A, Schweikert CH (1973) Experimentelle Untersuchungen über die elastische Druckverformung des Knochenschaftes. Z Orthop 111:791–795
Robinson R (1932) The significance of phosphoric ester in metabolism. New York University Press, New York
Röher O (1961) Die Bedeutung der Frequenz für Ultraschalltherapie. Dtsch Gesundh-Wesen 16:1943–1956
Schellnack K, Regling G, Regling S, Hähnel H, Trenschik K (1979) Elektrophysiologische Grundlagen der Fraktur- und Pseudarthrosenbehandlung durch Elektrostimulation. Beitr Orthop Traumatol 26:473–483
Schenk M, Kolb E (1982) Grundriß der physiologischen Chemie. Gustav Fischer, Jena
Schliephake E (1949) Anwendung von Ultraschall in der Medizin und Anwendung beim Gelenkrheumatismus. Strahlentherapie 79:613
Schneider UA, Steinemann S, Gueng W, Perren SM (1980) Die Belastung des Röhrenknochens mit programmierten dynamischen Kräften durch hydromechanische Implantate. Unfallheilkunde 83:173
Schubert T (1981) Fluoreszensmikroskopische Untersuchungen zum Einfluß von bipolaren Rechteckimpulsfolgen und dem Interferenzstromverhalten, Verfahren auf die Knochenbruchheilung – eine tierexperimentelle Studie. Dissertation, Medizinische Akademie Dresden
Schuster W et al. (1969) Quantitative Mineralsalzbestimmung am kindlichen Skelett. Dtsch Med Wochenschr 94:1983–1987
Schwarze E (1979) Kompendium der Veterinär-Anatomie, 3. Aufl. Bd 1. Gustav Fischer, Jena
Schweiberer L et al. (1973) Revascularisation der Tibia nach konservativer und operativer Frakturbehandlung. Hefte Unfallheilk 119:18–26
Segmüller G, Lech O, Bekier A (1969) Die osteogene Aktivität im Bereich der Pseudarthrose langer Röhrenknochen. Z Orthop 106:599–605
Strüter HD, Rassow J (1969) Über ein Verfahren zur quantitativen Bestimmung des Mineralgehaltes der Knochen mit radioaktiven Isotopen. Fortschr Röntgenstr 110:499–506
Stürmer KM, Schuchardt W (1980) Neue Aspekte der gedeckten Marknagelung und das Aufbohren der Markhöhle im Tierexperiment. Unfallheilkunde 83:341
Suzuki AK, Mathews A (1966) Two color fluorescent labelling of mineralizing tissues with tetracycline and 2,4 bis [N,N'-di-(carbomethyl)aminomethyl]fluorescein. Stain Technol 41:57–63
Trueta J (1974) Blood supply and the rate of healing of tibial fractures. Clin Orthop 105:11–17
Unterspann S, Finck W (1981) Untersuchungen zur Tc^{99m}Markierbarkeit von Derivaten der Aminomethandiphosphonsäure und zu ihrem Einsatz in der nuklearmedizinischen Skelettdiagnostik. Dtsch Gesundh-Wesen 36:2205–2210
Urist MR, Johnson RW (1943) Calcification and ossification. J Bone Joint Surg 25:375–426
Vinz H (1970) Die Änderung der Festigkeitseigenschaften des kompakten Knochengewebes im Laufe der Altersentwicklung. J Morph 115:257–272

Weigert M (1978) Der heutige Stand der Elektrostimulation der Knochenheilung beim Menschen. Z Orthop 116:600–601
Wehner W (1974) Die medizinische Bedeutung des Trennens und Schweißens von Knochen und anderen biologischen Geweben mit Ultraschall. Beitr Orthop Traumatol 21:648–650
Wiedau E, Röher D (1963) Ultraschall in der Medizin. Theodor Steinkopf, Dresden
Wolf E, Pompe B (1980) Rationelle und vereinfachte Kunststoffeinbettung mit Polymethakrylat für unentkalkte Knochenschnitte. Zentralbl Allg Pathol 124:551–556
Zichner L (1982) Vorgang der Kallusbildung unter Elektrostimulation, Z Orthop 120:441–442

Subject Index

absorption 41, 50
absorption coefficient 41, 44
alkaline phosphatase 69, 70, 80
–, levels 10
alternating acoustic pressure 41

bending strength 58, 80
blood flow improvement 25, 31, 33
bone index 13, 75
bone scintigraphy 10, 60–65, 82

calcaneal fractures 31
callus formation 1, 35, 36, 38, 54
–, delayed 3
cast window 4, 14, 18, 23, 25, 30, 31, 33
cavitation 43–45
clavicular fractures 24
continuous ultrasound 42
coupling, direct 4, 9, 14, 18, 23, 84
–, water immersion 4, 14, 17, 84

effects, biological 44
–, chemical 44
–, magnetostrictive 40
–, mechanical 43
–, physicochemical 44
–, thermal 44
electrical impedance 47
–, measurement 47f., 80

femoral fractures 29
fluorescence microscopy 78, 82
fluorochrome 77
fluorochrome uptake 77
forearm fractures 17

high-frequency instruments 81–84
high-frequency ultrasound 42
high-intensity ultrasound 43
humeral fractures 18

inorganic substances 71–75, 80
–, calcium 10, 68, 69, 73
–, carbon 68

–, copper 73
–, magnesium 68, 72
–, phosphorus 10, 68, 72
–, potassium 68, 73
–, sodium 68, 72
–, zinc 75
insonation, direct 4, 23–25, 30, 33
–, distant 4
–, dynamic 4, 9, 14, 18, 84
–, indirect 4
–, static 4, 84

low frequency 34, 35, 38
low-frequency instruments 31, 33, 85f.
low-frequency ultrasound 8, 42, 43

malleolar fractures 25
metacarpal fractures 14
metatarsal fractures 33
mineralization 54, 69, 80

nonunion 3
–, rate 13

patellar fractures 30
pH values 44, 80
–, measurement 70f.
phalangeal fractures 17
piezoelectric effect 1, 34, 40, 45, 49–51
–, reverse 40
proliferative activity 38
pulsed ultrasound 42

radial fractures 9–13
ROI activity quotient 10, 12, 63–65

scaphoid fractures 13f.
skin temperature, measurement 10, 13

temperature measurement 80
–, callus 80
–, rectal 79
tibial fractures 25, 54

total mineral content 10, 75
–, analysis 12, 75
trace elements 80
–, chlorine 68
–, copper 68
–, fluorine 68
–, iron 68
–, zinc 10, 68
transducer, large 4, 9
–, small 4, 14, 18, 23–25, 30, 31, 33

treatment, course 4, 9, 17, 18, 23–25, 29–33
–, duration 4, 9, 17, 18, 23, 24, 29, 31, 33

ultrasound absorption measurement 10, 13
ultrasound application *see* insonation
ultrasound conductivity 49
–, bone tissue 49
ultrasound frequency 38
ultrasound intensity 4, 9, 14, 17, 18, 23–25, 29–33, 36, 83
ultrasound therapy, contraindications 3
–, indications 3

vibration 34, 35, 41, 45
–, manual 35

wave length 38

G. Dagnini, Padova

Laparoscopy
and Imaging Techniques

With a Foreword by F. Vilardell

Translated from the Italian by S. Pearcey

1990. XI, 206 pp. 187 figs., 145 in color. 17 tabs.
Hardcover DM 298,- ISBN 3-540-50999-2

The value of laparoscopy as a diagnostic tool has changed dramatically in light of new, noninvasive imaging techniques. In this book a recognized expert gives an up-to-date account of the present uses of laparoscopy for the diagnosis of abdominal diseases. Although the indications for laparoscopy have radically changed, it still remains a viable and valuable diagnostic method. The author gives a complete discussion of technical innovations in laparoscopy and expertly evaluates its use. In particular he shows that, although this method has become redundant in some diseases, laparoscopy combined with sonography often gives the most complete diagnosis available today.
The step-by-step discussion and excellent endoscopic images make the book suitable for beginning laparoscopists. The general section covers new instruments and other technical innovations; the special section covers past and present indications; the remaining sections cover oncological laparoscopy and emergency laparoscopy.

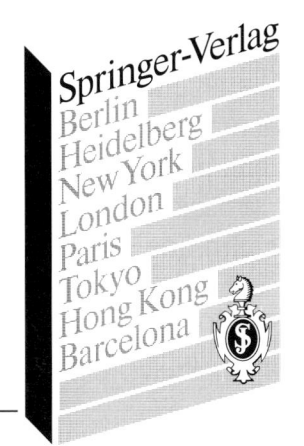

Springer-Verlag
Berlin
Heidelberg
New York
London
Paris
Tokyo
Hong Kong
Barcelona

Y. Higashi, Fukuoka University; Fukuoka
A. Mizushima, Kyushu University, Fukuoka;
H. Matsumoto, Okinawa, Japan

Introduction to Abdominal Ultrasonography

1991. XVI, 215 pp. 470 figs. Softcover DM 78,–
ISBN 3-540-51889-4

This book is designed specifically for residents in diagnostic radiology and those just beginning to undertake ultrasound diagnosis. Several features distinguish it from the monographs on ultrasound imaging of the abdomen that are already available. The clinical chapters begin with a detailed anatomical description of the organ or system. The most common diseases of the upper abdomen are presented, with each entity completely presented on two facing pages. The clinical discussions are brief and clear; the high-quality ultrasonograms are accompanied by schematic drawings and body marks for orientation and better understanding. A variety of different probes are presented: linear, sector, convex and contact compound. Particularly difficult imaging, for example the tubular structures of the liver, is supplemented with color illustrations to portray the three-dimensional quality of the actual examination.

The book also includes short chapters on basic physics, equipment, scanning technique and a question and answer section at the end.

Prices are subject to change without notice.

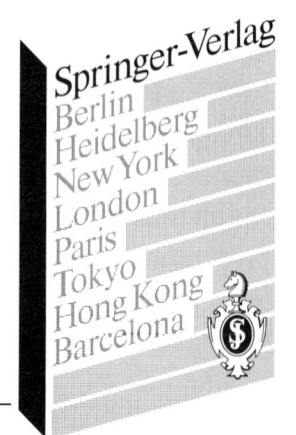